RAND NATIONAL DEFENSE RESEARCH INSTITUTE

T0146140

Integrating Department of Defense and Department of Veterans Affairs Purchased Care

Preliminary Feasibility Assessment

Carrie M. Farmer, Terri Tanielian, Christine Buttorff, Phillip Carter, Samantha Cherney, Erin L. Duffy, Susan D. Hosek, Lisa H. Jaycox, Ammarah Mahmud, Nicholas M. Pace, Lauren Skrabala, Christopher Whaley

Prepared for the Defense Health Agency and Veterans Health Administration

Approved for public release; distribution unlimited

For more information on this publication, visit www.rand.org/t/RR2762

Library of Congress Cataloging-in-Publication Data is available for this publication.
ISBN: 978-1-9774-0184-7

Published by the RAND Corporation, Santa Monica, Calif.
© Copyright 2018 RAND Corporation
RAND® is a registered trademark.

Limited Print and Electronic Distribution Rights

This document and trademark(s) contained herein are protected by law. This representation of RAND intellectual property is provided for noncommercial use only. Unauthorized posting of this publication online is prohibited. Permission is given to duplicate this document for personal use only, as long as it is unaltered and complete. Permission is required from RAND to reproduce, or reuse in another form, any of its research documents for commercial use. For information on reprint and linking permissions, please visit www.rand.org/pubs/permissions.

The RAND Corporation is a research organization that develops solutions to public policy challenges to help make communities throughout the world safer and more secure, healthier and more prosperous. RAND is nonprofit, nonpartisan, and committed to the public interest.

RAND's publications do not necessarily reflect the opinions of its research clients and sponsors.

Support RAND
Make a tax-deductible charitable contribution at
www.rand.org/giving/contribute

www.rand.org

Preface

The U.S. Department of Defense (DoD) and U.S. Department of Veterans Affairs (VA) are responsible for providing health care to eligible veterans, current and retired service members, and military dependents. DoD (through the TRICARE program) and VA (through the Veterans Health Administration, or VHA) provide a mix of care that is delivered at government-owned and -managed medical facilities ("direct care") and through private-sector contracts ("purchased care"). Through these purchased care contracts, third-party administrators (TPAs) coordinate and administer payments to community-based providers for delivering health care services to TRICARE beneficiaries or VHA enrollees. In the interest of expanding DoD-VA sharing, the DoD/VA Joint Executive Committee is exploring options to integrate DoD and VA's purchased care approaches (including contracting functions and provider networks) and asked the RAND Corporation to conduct a preliminary feasibility assessment of an integrated approach to purchasing care for the two departments.

To conduct the feasibility assessment, RAND reviewed relevant laws, regulations, and published literature; interviewed DoD and VA decisionmakers, congressional staff, and other stakeholders; and analyzed DoD and VA data on purchased care utilization and current TPA provider networks. This report describes the DoD and VA health care systems and current mechanisms for purchasing care, potential opportunities for joint purchasing of private care, and the legislative, policy, and operational challenges for integrating DoD and VA's approaches to purchasing care. The report also provides a cursory examination of the potential impact of an integrated purchased care contract on access, quality, and costs for beneficiaries and DoD/VA health systems.

This research was jointly sponsored by the Defense Health Agency and VHA and was conducted within the Forces and Resources Policy Center of the RAND National Defense Research Institute and the Payment, Cost, and Coverage Program in RAND Health Care.

The RAND National Defense Research Institute is a federally funded research and development center sponsored by the Office of the Secretary of Defense, the Joint Staff, the Unified Combatant Commands, the Navy, the Marine Corps, the defense agencies, and the defense Intelligence Community.

For more information on the RAND Forces and Resources Policy Center, see www.rand.org/nsrd/ndri/centers/frp or contact the director (contact information provided on the webpage).

RAND Health Care promotes healthier societies by improving health care systems in the United States and other countries. We do this by providing health care decisionmakers, practitioners, and consumers with actionable, rigorous, objective evidence to support their most complex decisions. For more information, see www.rand.org/health-care, or contact

RAND Health Care Communications
1776 Main Street
P.O. Box 2138
Santa Monica, CA 90407-2138
(310) 393-0411, ext. 7775
RAND_Health-Care@rand.org

Contents

Figures and Tables

Figures

Tables

Summary

The U.S. Department of Defense (DoD) and U.S. Department of Veterans Affairs (VA) operate large federal health systems serving distinct but sometimes overlapping populations of service members, veterans, and dependents. Both systems provide services through a mix of direct care, delivered at government-owned and -managed facilities, and purchased care, provided through the private sector, mainly by community-based providers who have entered into contracts with third-party administrators (TPAs). TPAs coordinate and administer reimbursements to network providers on behalf of DoD and VA for delivering health care services to eligible beneficiaries.

In the interest of expanding DoD-VA resource sharing to unlock greater efficiencies and cost savings, the DoD/VA Joint Executive Committee is exploring options to integrate DoD and VA's purchased care programs. DoD's Defense Health Agency (DHA) and VA's Veterans Health Administration (VHA) asked the RAND Corporation to conduct a preliminary feasibility assessment to determine how an integrated approach to purchasing care could affect access, quality, and costs for beneficiaries, DoD, and VA, as well as to identify general legislative, policy, or contractual challenges to implementing an integrated purchased care program.

Feasibility Assessment Scope and Methods

We examined whether the idea of an integrated approach to purchasing care was permissible under current legal and regulatory authority; feasible, given differences in how the two departments purchase care; and practical, given the operational missions of DoD and VA and the health care needs of the populations they serve. To address these questions, we explored the following factors that will have the greatest impact on feasibility:

- how current DoD and VA purchased care programs operate and the characteristics and health care needs of the populations they serve
- similarities and differences between DoD and VA purchased care contracts and how they compare to industry best practices
- the potential benefits and risks of an integrated purchased care approach for patients, DoD, and VA in terms of access, quality, patient experience, and costs
- legislative, policy, and operational opportunities and barriers.

Our assessment included a review of the published literature on private-sector and other government program practices for purchasing health care services. We also conducted interviews with DoD and VA officials who were responsible for overseeing the delivery of health care services and with representatives from TPAs and health benefits consulting firms, including individuals who have contracted with DoD or VA. We gathered additional feedback on potential barriers and facilitators to an integrated purchased care approach from representatives of military and veteran service organizations, as well as representatives from relevant congressional oversight committees. To help provide some historical context, we also spoke with individuals with expertise in the evolution of the TRICARE and VA purchased care programs.

Because there was not a shared understanding across stakeholders of what an integrated approach to purchasing care would look like, we assumed that such an approach would involve the two departments using a *single contract mechanism* to construct a shared network of health care providers who would serve the entire DoD and VA enrolled populations and that the new approach would involve some level of shared oversight by the two departments. We also assumed no changes to benefits (services offered/covered) or eligibility.

Overview of DoD and VA Health Care

Military Health System

DoD's Military Health System (MHS) provides care through the TRICARE program to 9.4 million eligible beneficiaries, including active-duty service members, reserve service members, retired military personnel, and their dependents. Services are delivered in military-owned treatment facilities or purchased from the private sector. In fiscal year (FY) 2017, the MHS provided direct care at 54 military hospitals and medical centers and 377 ambulatory clinics and employed more than 147,000 health care professionals, split between military and DoD civilian personnel (DoD, 2015). For active-duty beneficiaries, DoD purchases care from the private sector only when necessary to supplement military treatment facility (MTF) capacity (for example, when active-duty MTF personnel are deployed and capacity may be diminished).

Most other beneficiaries are required to enroll in one of two TRICARE plan options to receive care from the civilian sector: TRICARE Prime or TRICARE Select. Additional plans cover selected populations, such as those living abroad, retired reserve-component members and their families, and beneficiaries who are also eligible for Medicare. TRICARE benefits and plans differ slightly based on beneficiary category, although the differences are largely in how beneficiaries access care and their level of cost sharing. Active-duty military personnel pay no out-of-pocket costs for their health care. Family members of active-duty personnel do not pay out-of-pocket costs unless they use out-of-network care without a referral. Other beneficiaries pay enrollment fees and copayments, depending on their plan type and point of service (in-network or out-of-network provider).

DoD contracts with TPAs (also referred to as *managed care support contractors*) to manage and administer purchased care for the TRICARE program. Under the current TPAs, there are more than 570,000 community-based providers in the TRICARE network (DoD, 2015).

VA Health Care System

Through VHA, VA operates the largest integrated health care organization in the United States, with approximately 145 hospitals, more than 1,000 community-based outpatient clinics, 135 community living centers, 278 Vet Centers, and 48 domiciliaries (residential treatment programs) (VA, 2017a). In 2017, approximately 6.26 million veterans used VHA health care, out of approximately 9.05 million VHA-enrolled veterans (VA, 2017b) and nearly 20 million total veterans (Bagalman, 2014). In addition to providing health care for veterans, VHA also has education and research missions, providing training for physicians and other providers and developing new treatments for conditions common among veterans.

Modernizing VA health care has been a consistent theme throughout its history, and VA has gone through numerous transformations and reorganizations, many prompted by increases in the veteran population and the number and nature of benefits promised to service members.

Not all veterans are eligible for VA health care. Typically, veterans are eligible if they accumulate 24 consecutive months of active-duty service, separated under any condition other than dishonorable discharge, and have a health condition connected to their military service (VA, 2016b). However, there are some exceptions. For instance, some low-income veterans are eligible for VA care, as are some service members who have experienced military sexual trauma, even if they do not meet other VA eligibility requirements (VA, 2016b). In addition, certain veterans' dependents, caregivers, and survivors, as well as reservists who have served on active duty, are recognized as having veteran status. National Guard members activated in combat or a domestic emergency may also be eligible for VA benefits (Panangala, 2016; VA, 2016b).

VA health care is allocated based on the availability of resources (Panangala, 2016). Thus, eligibility is dependent on the department's budget. VA uses a "priority group" system to determine eligibility and resource allocation for groups of veterans. The priority group assignment is determined based on veterans' service-connected disabilities, income, service during a conflict, commendations, and other factors. Enrollees never pay for care for service-connected conditions, and copayments for non–service-connected conditions vary by priority group.

While VA has long purchased care from the private sector when it is unable to provide certain services through its medical facilities, the amount of VA purchased care has grown substantially in recent years. In FY 2014, VHA spent $6 billion on purchased care (Greenberg et al., 2015) and will spend an estimated $14.2 billion in FY 2019 (VA, 2019).

VA currently purchases care through a complex array of programs, including individual contracts with local providers (known as traditional purchased care) and contracts with TPAs to purchase care for large geographic regions. The TPAs administer two purchased care programs: the Patient-Centered Community Care (PC3) program and the Veterans Choice program. PC3 and Veterans Choice were established to address access issues that some veterans faced due to the unavailability of care from VA, veterans' geographic distance from a VA facility, or long wait times for an appointment. The VA Maintaining Systems and Strengthening Integrated Outside Networks (MISSION) Act, signed into law on June 6, 2018, consolidated these programs into one and created new authority for individual provider contracts, known as Veterans Care Agreements.

Patient Populations Served

A large proportion of the VA enrollee population is over age 65 (48 percent), whereas the TRICARE beneficiary population eligible to access the network is entirely under age 65. On the other end of the age range, there are no VA enrollees under age 18, while children make up 21 percent of the TRICARE beneficiary population. These significant age differences are important when considering the requirements of a joint purchased care contract, which would need to ensure the availability of care for the combined population of TRICARE beneficiaries and VA enrollees.

There are other differences in the two populations—including where they live (urban/rural) and their health care needs—that are critical to understand because these factors affect how a provider network under a joint purchased care contract would be designed and managed.

Roles of TPAs in DoD and VA

TPAs in the private sector generally take on a variety of administrative functions for employer-based health care plans. At a minimum, these functions include developing and maintaining provider networks and paying claims. TPAs can take on additional roles, such as developing benefit designs (which include the services covered and the associated cost sharing) and population health or utilization management activities.

The TPAs for TRICARE and VA currently have different roles because the nature of the types of care purchased differs greatly between the two departments. VA retains primary responsibility for patient care, referring patients to purchased care only for specific episodes of care, and, thus, almost all primary care is provided by VA providers in VA facilities. In contrast, TRICARE TPAs manage all of some TRICARE beneficiaries' care (e.g., for those enrolled in TRICARE Select), so primary care is provided through the TRICARE network rather than in MTFs. VA currently maintains more control over claims adjudication, while TRICARE requires that the TPAs take on this responsibility.

We examined differences in purchased care use between DoD and VA across nine types of care (inpatient, surgery, emergency care, primary care, physical therapies, oncology, obstetrics/gynecology, cardiology, and mental health care) and described each care type as a proportion of all purchased care visits or authorizations. Primary care makes up a large proportion (35 percent) of all purchased care visits for TRICARE but a very small proportion (3 percent) of VA purchased care authorizations.

Policy Implications, Conclusions, and Recommendations

Our review of the existing legal and regulatory authorities for DoD and VA indicated that an integrated purchased care approach (including a joint contract) would be legally permissible—with changes to existing authorities. Under current authorities and appropriations, each department could likely purchase care for its beneficiaries by adding the other department or its providers to its current contracts as subcontractors. Each department can also use its current appropriations to pay for its beneficiaries' care, if purchased through the programs described in those appropriations. However, notwithstanding the resource-sharing authorities, DoD and VA would likely need new statutory authority for a joint, integrated contract and would also likely need different appropriations language to purchase care through such a contract.

Over the past several years, there have been significant shifts in how both DoD and VA furnish health care, and both departments have been subject to congressionally mandated changes in how they manage and furnish health care. At the same time, the U.S. health care system has undergone changes that affect DoD and VA. Any decisions must consider how this evolving policy context will affect the feasibility and effectiveness of an integrated purchased care approach. For both departments, adapting to these policy changes has taken time and resources, and additional changes could disrupt ongoing efforts to implement the policy changes that are under way. Looking forward, both DoD and VA will need to prepare for uncertainty in demand for care that could result from changes to eligibility criteria or future combat operations. There is also uncertainty about the impact on patient experiences. Although our analysis confirmed that an integrated approach to purchasing care could expand the number of providers available to both departments, we were unable to determine whether this expansion would fill gaps for certain types of purchased care. Furthermore, without information about the capacity of each provider and the potential demand for their services under an integrated purchased care approach, it is difficult to assess the impact on patient access.

Our examination of costs also yielded uncertainty, as cost savings would depend on the extent to which DoD and VA harmonize their operational processes, including provider contracting, claims processing, reporting, and customer service functions. While some stakeholders believed that the government might be able to achieve greater cost-efficiency by negotiating lower payments to providers with an increased volume of services, both departments are already paying near Medicare rates to their contracted providers. To negotiate lower reimbursement rates, legislative change could be necessary—and doing so might have a negative impact on provider willingness to participate in a joint DoD/VA network. There could be some cost savings associated with integrating contracting functions and processes, but legal/regulatory changes in how those contracts are established would be required to achieve any real savings to the government (as opposed to merely shifting costs from one department to the other).

Recommendations

We offer two recommendations that are primarily aimed at reducing the uncertainty of the impact associated with an integrated purchased care approach. These recommendations should be considered in parallel but would likely best be implemented in sequence because the results of additional analysis will inform a demonstration or pilot and provide the most concrete evidence of impact on the dimensions of interest.

Conduct Additional Analyses

To gain a more robust understanding of whether merging provider networks would help improve provider access, it is necessary to identify similarities and differences in demand for purchased care using individual-level data, as well as data on specific regions and patient populations. It will also be necessary to determine whether providers perceive barriers to participating as the network of one department versus the other to understand whether providers would want to join this joint network. Further analyses on merging contracting functions could also explore specific staffing capabilities and needs across DoD and VA, as well as various options for joint oversight, their advantages and disadvantages, and their costs.

Design, Implement, and Evaluate a Pilot or Demonstration Project

Establishing an integrated purchased care program would take several years, but a series of pilots or demonstrations, perhaps focused on a specific type of service, could help clarify how integration might affect access, costs, and quality of care and pave the way to full integration later on. Prior experiences with resource sharing between DoD and VA offer potential insights for these demonstrations.

Acknowledgments

We are grateful to the many individuals who helped facilitate this study, including the DHA and VHA staffs who provided access to the information used in our analyses. We also acknowledge the support and assistance of our project monitors, Patrick Grady (DHA), Gene Migliaccio (VHA), and Brady White (VHA). We thank the stakeholders who participated in our interviews, including those from military and veteran support organizations, congressional oversight committees, and federal staffs in both DoD and VA. Without their input, much of the analyses presented in this report would not have been possible. We are grateful for the research support from Laura Pavlock-Albright, Simon Hollands, and Amy Grace Donohue. We also thank our technical peer reviewers, Kenneth Kizer, Andrew Mulcahy, and Jeanne Ringel. Their constructive comments and feedback helped us improve and refine our analyses, as well as clarify this report.

Abbreviations

ACA	Affordable Care Act
ACO	accountable care organization
CAHPS	Consumer Assessment of Healthcare Providers and Systems
C.F.R.	Code of Federal Regulations
CHAMPVA	Civilian Health and Medical Program of the Department of Veterans Affairs
CMS	Centers for Medicare and Medicaid Services
DFARS	Defense Federal Acquisition Regulation Supplement
DHA	Defense Health Agency
DoD	U.S. Department of Defense
EHR	electronic health record
FAR	Federal Acquisition Regulation
FTE	full-time equivalent
FY	fiscal year

HEDIS	Healthcare Effectiveness Data and Information Set
HMO	health maintenance organization
MCSC	managed care support contractor
MERHCF	Medicare-Eligible Retiree Health Care Fund
MHS	Military Health System
MTF	military treatment facility
OB/GYN	obstetrics/gynecology
OSD	Office of the Secretary of Defense
PC3	Patient-Centered Community Care
PPBE	Planning, Programming, Budgeting, and Execution
PPO	preferred provider organization
RFP	request for proposal
TFL	TRICARE for Life
TPA	third-party administrator
U.S.C.	U.S. Code
VA	U.S. Department of Veterans Affairs
VAAR	Veterans Affairs Acquisition Supplement
VAMC	VA medical center
VA MISSION Act	VA Maintaining Systems and Strengthening Integrated Outside Networks Act of 2018
VFW	Veterans of Foreign Wars
VHA	Veterans Health Administration

CHAPTER ONE

Background

The U.S. Department of Defense (DoD) and U.S. Department of Veterans Affairs (VA) each operate large federal health systems, serving distinct but overlapping populations. Across the two departments, health care is provided to eligible veterans, current and retired service members, and military dependents. Each of these systems was constructed with different primary missions, however, and each has evolved substantially over the past 30 years. DoD and VA provide health care through a mix of care that is delivered at government-owned and -managed medical facilities (*direct care*) and care that is provided through the private sector (*purchased care*). Much of the care purchased from the private sector is obtained from community-based providers who have entered into contracts with third-party administrators (TPAs) on behalf of DoD or VA to be a part of their respective health care networks. Through these contracts, TPAs coordinate and administer payments to providers for delivering health care services to individuals who are eligible to receive health care benefits from DoD or VA. In the interest of expanding efforts to share resources (e.g., capabilities, expertise, facilities) across DoD and VA and to create potential operational efficiencies, the DoD/VA Joint Executive Committee is exploring options to integrate DoD and VA's purchased care approaches (including contracting and provider networks).[1]

---

[1] 10 U.S.C. 1096 gives DoD this authority:

> The Secretary of Defense may enter into an agreement providing for the sharing of resources between facilities of the uniformed services and facilities of a civilian health care provider or providers that the Secretary contracts with under section 1079, 1086, or

In early 2018, the Defense Health Agency (DHA) and the Veterans Health Administration (VHA) asked the RAND Corporation to carry out a preliminary feasibility assessment to consider the effect of an integrated approach to purchasing care on operational efficiency as well as the potential effect on access, quality, and costs for beneficiaries, DoD, and VA. DHA and VHA also asked RAND to begin to identify legislative, policy, or contractual challenges the departments would face in implementing an integrated purchased care program. This report presents the findings from that assessment.

Scope and Methods of Feasibility Assessment

Feasibility assessments typically examine the practicality of a proposed plan or method and attempt to answer the question, "Can it work?" (Bowen et al., 2009). In the business sector, a feasibility assessment is often conducted to determine whether a plan or product (1) is technically feasible, (2) is feasible within the estimated costs, and (3) will be profitable. Often, the feasibility assessment is guided by a sense of the amount of resources and time available to implement said plan. More broadly, this type of assessment can be used to examine whether a suggested method or plan is possible or reasonable, given current laws or regulations, as well as the operational and technical capabilities available to the organization(s).

For our purposes, we examined whether an integrated purchased care approach (including a joint purchased care contract) was permissible under current legal and regulatory authority, feasible given differences in how DoD and VA purchase care currently, and practical given the operational missions of the two departments and the health care needs of populations they serve.

To conduct the preliminary feasibility assessment, we examined

---

1097 of this title if the Secretary determines that such an agreement would result in the delivery of health care to which covered beneficiaries are entitled under this chapter in a more effective, efficient, or economical manner.

- current DoD and VA purchased care programs, as well as the characteristics and health care needs of their relevant covered populations
- similarities and differences between DoD and VA purchased care contracts and comparisons to industry best practices
- the potential impact (advantages and disadvantages) of an integrated purchased care approach on covered populations, DoD, and VA in terms of access, quality, patient experience, and costs
- legislative, policy, and operational facilitators and barriers.

Data Sources

We relied on various sources of information. We reviewed and extracted insights and data points from published reports on DoD and VA health care and published literature on private-sector and other government program practices for purchasing health care services. We also relied on insights and expertise gathered from stakeholders and others with expertise in these topics. To this end, we conducted interviews with officials within both departments. We spoke primarily with those in positions responsible for overseeing the delivery of health care services across the direct and purchased care programs. We also spoke with representatives from TPAs and health benefit consulting firms, including those who are currently or have formerly contracted with DoD, VA, or both. We gathered feedback on the potential barriers and facilitators to an integrated purchased care approach from representatives in military and veteran service organizations, as well as representatives from the relevant congressional oversight committees. To help provide some historical context, we also spoke with individuals with expertise on the evolution of the TRICARE and VA purchased care programs. In total, we spoke with 39 individuals across these groups.

We also requested and reviewed aggregated data on purchased care utilization from both DoD and VA over the past two years. We used these data to describe the volume and type of care that each department purchases from the private sector. We reviewed the existing contract documents that DoD and VA use to manage their relationships with the TPAs that are responsible for administering their purchased care programs. We also reviewed the new requests for proposals (RFPs) from VA for its next contracting period, and we assessed similarities and differences across key functions of TPAs that are common in the private sector. Additionally, we compared the common private-sector practices in key domains, as well as other domains that may be included in the contracts in the future.

To examine how the current DoD and VHA purchased care provider networks compare, we combined data from several sources into a provider-level data set on all providers currently in either the DoD or VA network. We obtained provider spreadsheets from DHA and VHA with a detailed coding of provider specialty and office address, including zip code, and used data from the U.S. Census Bureau to describe beneficiary populations at the county level.

To assess legislative and policy issues arising from this proposed plan, we reviewed the legal authorities for DoD and VA contained in Titles 10 and 38, respectively, of the U.S. Code, as well as general fiscal law and contracting authorities contained in Titles 31 and 41 of the U.S. Code. We also reviewed appropriations laws for DoD and VA, focusing on provisions related to health care. Alongside these authorities, we examined legislative reports accompanying recent TRICARE and VA purchased care legislation, including both authorizing and appropriations legislation. We also reviewed relevant policies and regulations, including the Federal Acquisition Regulation (FAR), the Defense Federal Acquisition Regulation Supplement (DFARS), the Veterans Affairs Acquisition Regulation (VAAR), and agency policies and directives relating to purchased care. Our project was reviewed by RAND's Human Subjects Protection Committee and determined not to be human subjects research.

Framing the Feasibility Study

Early in the study, it became clear that different stakeholders had different views of what integration of purchased care approaches might entail. For example, in discussing the design of a joint purchased care contract, many interviewees implied that they believed that both DoD military treatment facilities (MTFs) and VA facilities would be among the list of available network providers. In other words, VA hospitals and clinics could see TRICARE beneficiaries who were not already enrolled in VA and vice versa (veterans could go to MTFs without being enrolled in TRICARE Prime). There was a general supposition that a move in this direction could ultimately benefit the patient in terms of continuity of care across the lifespan and round out health care services available through the purchased care networks. However, there were also concerns about the capacity of each of the government-owned facilities to accommodate potential demand from the other beneficiary group, and about the need to make adjustments to comple-ment—rather than duplicate—each other in terms of expertise and capacity.

An integrated approach to purchasing care could be more or less complex than the present situation, depending on the specifics of how DoD and VA would work together and how integrated the two health care systems would become. Because there was a not a shared under-standing of what integrating purchased care would mean, we made some assumptions about what a future integrated purchased care approach would entail and used those assumptions to guide our assess-ment. Based on discussions with our project sponsors about the dimen-sions of an integrated purchased care approach, we assumed that DoD and VA would use a *single contract mechanism* that engages TPAs to construct a *network of health care providers that would serve the entire DoD and VHA enrolled populations* and that would involve some level of *shared oversight by DoD and VA*. In examining the feasibility of an integrated purchased care approach, we assumed no changes to ben-efits (services offered/covered) or eligibility for either program. We also assumed no major changes in demand. We note, however, that during our feasibility assessment, legislative changes were passed that will affect eligibility for VHA's purchased care program. We reviewed pro-posed changes at the time of our analysis and took them into account as best we could.

In addition to varying views of what integration might entail, there were varying levels of understanding of the respective health care systems among the stakeholders we interviewed. Many interviewees revealed that they did not understand how the other system worked, with VA staff expressing some confusion about TRICARE and vice versa. This was particularly an issue with respect to understanding how individuals access health care services—for example, who was eligible for what types of health benefits and how one would access health care in the private sector. A few interviewees, however, had worked across systems or received medical care in a different system from the one in which they worked, and they were able to compare some aspects of their experiences (such as appointment scheduling and quality of care) directly. We therefore begin this report with an overview of the two systems to put all readers on the same footing in evaluating the possibility of integration.

Organization of This Report

Chapter Two provides some basic information about these federal health systems, including information on who they serve, how they are organized, and how their purchased care programs fit within the larger system of care. Chapter Three provides a more detailed comparison of how DoD and VA use purchased care, including a detailed breakdown of utilization and a comparison of existing provider networks. Chapter Four reviews the legal and regulatory authorities that pertain to integration. Chapter Five describes various aspects related to operational execution of an integrated purchased care approach and Chapter Six summarizes perspectives about the potential impact that integration would have on access, quality, and beneficiary experiences. Chapter Seven describes cost considerations that need further exploration. Finally, in Chapter Eight, we summarize the findings and make recommendations for moving forward.

CHAPTER TWO

Overview of DoD and VA Health Care

There are three main sectors in which service members, veterans, and their families may seek health care services:

- the MHS, operated by DoD
- the VA health care system, operated by VHA
- the rest of the U.S. health care system.

Both the MHS and the VA health care system provide a mix of direct care (i.e., care provided in government-owned and -managed facilities, including through MTFs and VHA medical centers, respectively) and purchased care (i.e., care paid for by the MHS or VHA but delivered by private, community-based providers). These three sectors serve overlapping populations of military personnel, veterans, and their families, some of whom may be eligible for care in more than one sector at the same time. Furthermore, the range of eligibility requirements and health care options affects how patients use their health care coverage options. For example, the majority of veterans are also covered by Medicare, Medicaid, or private health insurance plans, and some DoD beneficiaries also have other forms of health coverage. While most family members are not eligible for direct VA care, some are eligible for VA purchased care benefits, for example, through CHAMPVA (Civilian Health and Medical Program of the Department of Veterans Affairs).[1] This chapter provides

---

[1] Veteran family members may be eligible for counseling at Vet Centers or for benefits through CHAMPVA, the Foreign Medical Program, Children of Women Vietnam Veterans Program, Spina Bifida Healthcare Program, and the Caregiver Program.

a brief description of the MHS and the VA health care system based largely on publicly available information from both departments.

Military Health System

Through its TRICARE program, the MHS covers 9.4 million eligible beneficiaries, including active-duty service members, reserve service members, retired military personnel, and their dependents through services delivered in military-owned treatment facilities and those purchased from the private sector. There are two main types of MHS beneficiaries: sponsors (active-duty, retired, and National Guard/reserve service members) and their family members (spouses and dependents who are registered in the Defense Enrollment Eligibility Reporting System) (TRICARE, 2016).

MHS Mission and Organization

The MHS has a three-part mission:

> (1) to ensure America's 1.3 million active duty and 1.1 million reserve-component personnel are healthy so they can complete their national security missions; (2) to ensure that all active and reserve medical personnel in uniform are trained and ready to provide medical care in support of operational forces around the world, and (3) to provide a medical benefit commensurate with the service and sacrifice of more than 9.4 million active duty personnel, military retirees and their families. (MHS, undated[a])

To achieve these missions, the MHS works in multiple areas, including health care delivery, medical education, private-sector partnerships, and medical research and development (MHS, undated[d]). To deliver health care services, MHS relies on the TRICARE program to deliver both direct care (delivered in MTFs) and purchased care (delivered by private-sector providers), with expenditures split roughly in half between the two (DoD, 2015)

Direct care is provided at MTFs, mostly located on military installations and in areas that are densely populated by TRICARE beneficiaries (see Figure 2.1). In fiscal year (FY) 2017, the MHS provided direct care at 54 military hospitals and medical centers and 377 ambulatory clinics, and it employed more than 147,000 health care professionals, split between military and DoD civilian personnel (DoD, 2015). Active-duty service members are required to seek non-emergency health care at military hospitals or clinics if possible (TRICARE, 2016). If such services are not available, active-duty service members must get a referral from a primary care manager before care from a community-based provider will be covered (TRICARE, 2016).

Figure 2.1
MHS Facilities and Size of the TRICARE Beneficiary Population, by County

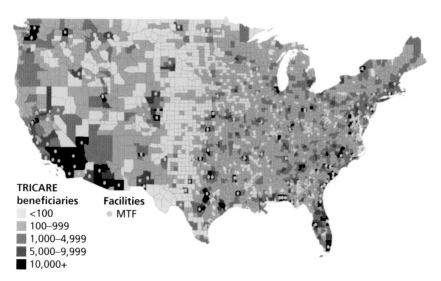

SOURCES: Defense Medical Information System data on MTF locations as of FY 2017. County population data come from the U.S. Census Bureau's American Fact Finder county-level tables, which are derived from the full sample of the 2012–2016 American Community Survey. The household respondent is asked to describe each household member's health insurance coverage. Respondents may report more than one type of insurance, so individuals reporting both VA and TRICARE coverage are likely to be double-counted in the Census Bureau's tables.

DoD Purchased Care

DoD supplements the MTF capabilities with care purchased from the private sector through provider networks established and managed by contractors known as TPAs.[2] For the purposes of organizing and delivering care through these TPAs, TRICARE is split into two geographic regions. DoD relies on the TRICARE network to provide one-third of its ongoing health care services for dependents of active-duty service members and most services for retirees and their dependents (TRICARE, 2018b).

TRICARE was named for its original offering of three types of insurance packages: TRICARE Prime (structured like a health maintenance organization, or HMO), TRICARE Standard (a traditional fee-for-service option), and TRICARE Extra (a preferred provider network option added to TRICARE Standard). Purchased care, as in care bought from the civilian sector, is paid for as a typical insurer-to-provider arrangement without DoD employing the provider. Beginning in 2018, DoD consolidated TRICARE into two basic options: TRICARE Prime and TRICARE Select, which combined TRICARE Standard and TRICARE Extra to form a preferred provider organization (PPO). Beneficiaries are required to enroll in one of these plans to receive care from the civilian sector. Under the current TPAs, there are more than 570,000 network providers (DoD, 2015). Additional plans—beyond the basic two—cover selected populations, such as those living abroad and reserve-component members and their families. TRICARE for Life (TFL), for example, provides Medicare wraparound coverage for beneficiaries who are entitled to Medicare.

Congress appropriates an account of funds each year to DoD for the Defense Health Program, a component of which is the TRICARE program. In its Consolidated Appropriations Act for 2018, Congress appropriated $34.4 billion for the Defense Health Program, "of which $15,349,700,000 may be available for contracts entered into under the TRICARE program" (Pub. L. 115-141, 2018, Title VI, Div. C). The Defense Health Program account funds most of the Unified Medical Program, a $54 billion program that includes all defense health

---

[2]   Within DoD, these TPAs are referred to as managed care support contractors (MCSCs).

programs (including amounts spent on MTFs and military medical personnel). In addition to the annual appropriations from Congress that fund the Unified Medical Program, DoD uses the Medicare-Eligible Retiree Health Care Fund (MERHCF) to pay "the cost of DoD health care programs (both direct and purchased care) for Medicare-eligible retirees, retirees' family members, and survivors" (DoD, 2018, pp. 27–28). In 2017 and 2018, DoD estimated that it would receive approximately $10.4 billion from the MERHCF to pay for care for retirees and their dependents.

There are different eligibility requirements for each of the TRICARE programs (see Table 2.1). Individuals who are eligible for TRICARE Prime are active-duty service members, their dependents, and survivors. Survivors are spouses, dependents, and unmarried persons under the legal custody of service members who died while on active duty for 30 or more days.[3] Also eligible for Prime are

> retirees, dependents of retirees, and survivors who are not eligible for Medicare Part A based on age . . . in locations where it is offered and where an MTF has, in the judgment of the Director, a significant number of health care providers, including specialty care providers, and sufficient capability to support the efficient operation of TRICARE Prime for projected retired beneficiary enrollees in that location. (32 C.F.R. 199.17[c])[4]

The individuals who are eligible for TRICARE Select are dependents and survivors of active-duty service members[5] and "all retirees, dependents of retirees, and survivors who are not eligible for Medicare Part A" (32 C.F.R. 199.17[c]). Also eligible are "member[s] of the

---

[3] Survivors are eligible for TRICARE Prime for three years after the service member's death or, for dependents and unmarried persons under the service member's legal custody, until they reach 21 years old or stop pursuing full-time education by age 23 (if they had been doing so at age 21) and were dependent on the service member for more than half of their support at the time of the service member's death (32 C.F.R. 199.17[c]).

[4] Medicare Part A, which is hospital insurance, is offered to individuals age 65 and older (Centers for Medicare and Medicaid Services [CMS], 2015).

[5] If they reside in areas where TRICARE Prime is not offered (32 C.F.R. 199.17[c]).

Table 2.1
Overview of TRICARE Plans for Eligible Beneficiaries

Program	Eligibility	Design	Access	Cost Sharing
TRICARE Prime	Active-duty military (including activated reservists) and their families	HMO with primary care and specialty care from military or contracted civilian providers	Beneficiaries must use their Prime provider for services or face cost sharing if they seek care from non-Prime providers without a referral.	No cost
	Retirees (generally with 20+ years of service) and their dependents; medical retirees	HMO with primary care from military or contracted civilian providers.	Beneficiaries must use their Prime provider for services or face cost sharing if they seek care from non-Prime providers without a referral.	Enrollment fee and copayments for in-network care; deductibles and coinsurance for out-of-network care
TRICARE Select	Active-duty dependents, retirees and dependents (up to age 65)	Fee for service with care from MTFs or civilian providers; reduced cost sharing when participants use contracted providers; similar to a PPO	Beneficiaries can choose which provider they seek care from in the private sector but face different cost sharing, depending on whether they see a network provider or an out-of-provider.	Enrollment fee for retirees and dependents; copay schedule for in-network care; deductible and coinsurance for out-of-network care
TFL	Medicare-enrolled retirees and dependents	Medicare wraparound	Beneficiaries seek care from Medicare providers.	Services covered by TRICARE but not by Medicare are subject to deductible and coinsurance

Selected Reserve of the Ready Reserve of a reserve component,"[6] their dependents, and survivors for the period of service;[7] members of the retired reserve of a reserve component who qualify for a non-regular retirement at age 60 under 10 U.S.C. 1223 but are not yet age 60,[8] their dependents, and survivors.[9] Service members are eligible only until they become eligible for other TRICARE coverage at age 60 (10 U.S.C. 1076e), this coverage is not available to those who are eligible for health insurance for government employees under Title 5, Chapter 89, of the U.S. Code, , and it carries a substantially higher premium contribution than the other TRICARE plans (10 U.S.C. 1076e; 5 U.S.C. 89). Finally, TRICARE Select is also offered to children who would be considered dependent but are older than 21 but under age 26, are not otherwise eligible for an employee-sponsored health care plan, and are not dependents of any other service member or former service member (Miles, 2011).[10]

As noted earlier, TFL eligibility extends to TRICARE beneficiaries with Medicare Part A and B. According to the TFL handbook, the following individuals who are eligible for Medicare Part A, hospital insurance, must also enroll in Medicare Part B, medical insurance, to remain TRICARE-eligible: retirees, their family members, survivors, eligible former spouses, and Medal of Honor recipients and eligible family members (TRICARE, 2018a).

TRICARE benefits and plans differ slightly by beneficiary category, although the differences are largely in how beneficiaries access care and their level of cost sharing (TRICARE, 2016). Active-duty military personnel pay no out-of-pocket costs for their health care.

---

[6] This is called TRICARE Reserve Select (10 U.S.C. 1075, 1076d).

[7] Survivors are eligible for six months after the death of the service member (10 U.S.C. 1076d).

[8] This is called TRICARE Retired Reserve (10 U.S.C. 1075, 1076e).

[9] Survivors are eligible for six months after the death of the service member (10 U.S.C. 1076e).

[10] This is known as the TRICARE Young Adult program (10 U.S.C. 1075, 1110b). This provision was added so that military families would be offered the same coverage for unmarried dependent children as families under the ACA.

Family members of active-duty personnel do not have out-of-pocket costs unless they use out-of-network care without a referral. Other beneficiaries pay enrollment fees and copayments, depending on their plan type and point of service (in-network or out-of-network provider).

It should be noted that TRICARE beneficiaries can access any private, community-based provider they choose. However, whether the services will be (or to what extent they would be) paid for by TRICARE varies based on the plan in which the patient is enrolled and whether the provider is part of the TRICARE network. For example, a TRICARE Prime enrollee could seek care from a private-sector provider, but TRICARE would pay for those services only if a Prime provider made the referral.

VA Health Care System

VA, through VHA, operates the largest integrated health care organization in the United States, with approximately 145 medical centers, more than 800 community-based outpatient clinics, 135 community living centers, 278 Vet Centers, and 48 domiciliaries (residential treatment programs) (VA, 2017a). Contrary to common understanding, fewer than half of U.S. military veterans are eligible for VA health care. Eligibility for VA health care is based on length of service, having a service-connected health condition, income, and other factors. In 2017, approximately 6.26 million veterans used VHA health care, out of approximately 9.05 million VHA-enrolled veterans for that year (VA, 2017b) and a total population of nearly 20 million veterans (Bagalman, 2014).

Government-provided support for disabled veterans dates back to the American Revolution, although at that time it consisted primarily of pensions for seriously disabled veterans or their survivors (Severo and Milford, 1989; Rostker, 2013). From the Revolution through the Civil War, individual states and communities provided direct medical and hospital care to injured and disabled soldiers. State homes, many of which offered domiciliary care, were established after the Civil War. The facilities were designed primarily to serve indigent and disabled veterans, although some service members also received care in these homes. In 1865, President Abraham Lincoln signed a law to establish a national asylum for soldiers and sailors. It was renamed the National Home for Disabled Volunteer Soldiers in 1873, but it only served soldiers who fought in the Union Army. World War I brought the establishment of a national system of veterans' hospitals. To create this system, the Bureau of War Risk Insurance and the Public Health Service leased hundreds of private hospitals and hotels for the rush of returning injured war veterans and began a program of building new hospitals. Oversight of these systems was consolidated under the Veterans Administration in 1930 (this consolidation also included the Bureau of Pensions), uniting, for the first time, health care and benefit programs for veterans under a single entity at the federal level.

Modernizing VA has been a consistent theme throughout its history. As a federal entity, VA has gone through numerous transformations and reorganizations, many of them prompted by growth in the size of the veteran population and the number and nature of benefits promised to service members. VA was established as a federal Cabinet-level department in 1989, and VA's Department of Medicine and Surgery (established in 1946) became VHA in 1991, one of the three main components of the department (the other two being the Veterans Benefits Administration and the National Cemetery Administration).

The Veterans' Health Care Eligibility Reform Act of 1996 changed eligibility requirements and enrollment processes for veterans, with the dual effects of increasing access to VA health care for many veterans and tiering this access into a system of priority groups based on service-connected disability status, military service, and income, among other factors (Pub. L. 104-262, 110 Stat. 3177; 38 U.S.C. 1705). This tiered priority group system exists in largely the same form today (VA, 2016c). In the mid-1990s, VA also restructured its health care system into the current network of hospitals, clinics, and regional VA Integrated Service Networks (VISNs) (Kizer, Demakis, and Feussner, 2000; Kizer and Dudley, 2009).

VHA Mission and Organization

VHA's mission is to "honor America's Veterans by providing exceptional health care that improves their health and well-being." To fulfill this mission, VHA provides a full array of direct health care treatments and services to eligible veterans, executes a very large research program, and hosts multiple training opportunities (e.g., residencies, clinical internships) for health professionals. VHA provides most health care through VA-owned and -operated medical centers and outpatient clinics, and it purchases care from the community/private sector only when necessary.

As noted, not all veterans are eligible for VA health care. Typically, veterans are eligible for VA health care if they accumulate 24 consecutive months of active-duty military service, separated under any condition other than dishonorable discharge, and have a health condition connected to their military service (VA, 2016b). However, there are some exceptions. For instance, in certain cases, low-income veterans may be eligible for VA care. Service members who have experienced military sexual trauma are eligible for VA health care to address health needs related to military sexual trauma incidents, even if they do not meet other VA eligibility requirements (VA, 2016b). In addition, certain veterans' dependents, caregivers, and survivors are eligible for CHAMPVA, which functions like an insurance program by reimbursing private providers and facilities for beneficiaries' medical care (Panangala, 2016). Reservists who have served on active duty are recognized as having veteran status and may be eligible for VA benefits, and National Guard members may also be eligible for VA benefits if they have been activated for federal service (VA, 2016b). However, reservists and National Guard members have limited eligibility for VA health care if they have not experienced full-time activation for federal service.

VA health care is allocated based on the availability of resources (Panangala, 2016). Thus, VA health care eligibility depends on the department's budget. VA uses a "priority group" system to determine eligibility and resource allocation for groups of veterans. Priority group assignments are determined based on veterans' service-connected disabilities, income, service during a conflict, commendations, and other factors. Enrollees never pay for care for service-connected conditions, and some priority groups have copayments for non–service-connected conditions. The system was legislated in the mid-1990s to help VHA ensure that those who would have the need for VHA would be given priority access (Pub. L. 104-262, 110 Stat. 3177; 38 U.S.C. 1705). At present, as mentioned, the priority group system uses a mix of criteria, including level of disability and income, to assign enrollees to one of eight groups.[11] Special exceptions have been made to increase access to VA health care for veterans who have recently returned from combat. Within five years of discharge, post-9/11 veterans are eligible to enroll in VA health care without needing to prove that their illness or injury is service-connected and without having to meet an income requirement (Panangala, 2016). Once veterans enroll in VA care under the extended eligibility authority, they may continue receiving health care beyond the five-year eligibility period (Panangala, 2016).

In mid-2017, the VA Secretary announced plans to make some mental health services available to veterans with other-than-honorable discharges. This policy change was largely motivated by concerns that many of these individuals could have qualified for a medical discharge, as well as the increased rates of homelessness and suicide among veterans with other-than-honorable discharge status. On July 5, 2017, these veterans became eligible for VA emergency mental health services. As of this writing, it is not known how this policy change will affect demand for these services and their use or how VHA will meet the longer-term mental health needs of this population.

Family members are not eligible to enroll in the VA health system; however, some dependents and survivors are eligible to receive certain reimbursements. For example, primary caregivers who are uninsured can receive training, counseling, and mental health services through the Program of Comprehensive Support for Caregivers.

Most veterans who are enrolled in VA health care have other sources of health coverage (e.g., Medicare, TRICARE, employer-sponsored insurance) and use VA to meet, on average, 30 percent of

---

[11] The current distribution of enrollees by priority group is highlighted in Figure 2.5, along-side a discussion of the populations served by both departments

their health care needs (Eibner et al., 2015). Enrolled veterans make decisions about whether to use VA or other health coverage based on access, perceived quality, out-of-pocket costs, and other factors. When these factors change—for example, when some veterans became eligible for other health insurance under the Affordable Care Act (ACA)—reliance on VA health care, or the proportion of care that enrolled veterans receive from VA relative to other health coverage, changes as well (Dworsky et al., 2017).

VHA operates 172 large medical centers (called VAMCs) and more than 1,000 community-based outpatient clinics through 21 VISNs. VHA uses the VISN model to oversee its clinical assets. As shown in Figure 2.2, VA clinical facilities are geographically distributed across the United States.

Figure 2.2
VA Facilities and Size of the VA Enrollee Population, by County

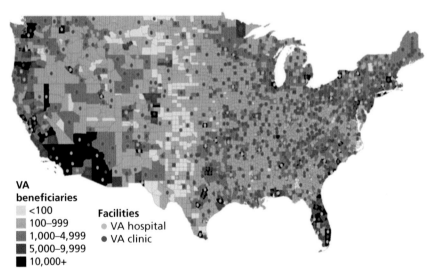

SOURCES: VA data on facility locations as of FY 2017. County population data come from the U.S. Census Bureau's American Fact Finder county-level tables, which are derived from the full sample of the 2012–2016 American Community Survey. The household respondent is asked to describe each household member's health insurance coverage. Respondents may report more than one type of insurance, so individuals reporting both VA and TRICARE coverage are likely to be double-counted in the Census Bureau's tables.

VHA Purchased Care

While VA has long purchased care from the private sector when it is unable to provide certain services through its medical facilities, in recent years, the amount of VA purchased care has grown substantially. In FY 2014, VHA spent $6 billion on purchased care (Greenberg et al., 2015); in its FY 2019 budget request, VA estimated purchased care costs of $14.2 billion (VA, 2019).

VA purchases care through a complex array of programs, including individual contracts with local providers (known as traditional purchased care) and contracts with TPAs to purchase care for large geographic regions (see Figure 2.3). The TPAs administer two purchased care programs: the Patient-Centered Community Care (PC3) program and the Veterans Choice program. PC3 and Veterans Choice were established to address access issues that some veterans faced due to the unavailability of care from VA, veterans' geographic distance from a VA facility, or long wait times for an appointment. PC3 was originally established in 2012 to provide additional VA capacity for specialty care. In 2014, Congress passed the Veterans Access to Care Through Choice, Accountability, and Transparency Act in response to an outcry about veterans facing long wait times for care and a scandal involving the falsification of wait-time data. The act established the Veterans Choice program to serve veterans living more than 40 miles from a VA facility or waiting longer than 30 days for an appointment. It also required VA to implement the Veterans Choice program within 90 days. To meet the implementation deadline without having to build and compete a new large contract, existing PC3 contracts were modified to add the Veterans Choice components. The VA Maintaining Internal Systems and Strengthening Integrated Outside Networks (MISSION) Act, signed into law on June 6, 2018, consolidates these programs into one and creates new authority for individual provider contracts that are now called Veterans Care Agreements (38 U.S.C. 1703A, as amended).

Not all VHA-enrolled veterans are eligible to receive care in the community. If VA is unable to provide specific, required health care services to an enrolled veteran patient (due to, for example, insufficient capacity or capabilities), it will authorize the purchase of that specific

Figure 2.3
VA Purchased Care Programs

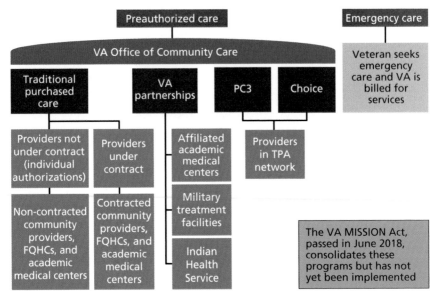

NOTE: FQHC = federally qualified health center.

care from the private sector through one of its existing contract mechanisms. Only that episode of care is then authorized to be purchased in the private sector. VHA enrollees who are eligible for purchased care *do* have a choice with respect to whom they seek care from in the community; however, they must work with the TPA or with VHA to ensure that the provider is eligible to receive payments from VHA.

With the passage of the VA MISSION Act, VA has one year to establish new eligibility criteria for purchased care that consider patient preference and the quality of care available from a veteran's assigned VA facility.

MHS and VHA Populations

This section provides an overview of the size and characteristics of the populations served by the MHS and VHA.

MHS Users

Approximately 9.4 million individuals are eligible for DoD health care (TRICARE, 2017). This number has been relatively stable over the past several years, although there have been slight shifts in the size of the population by beneficiary group. Since the end of the Cold War, the number of active-duty personnel has decreased by one-third, and the number of living retirees eligible for TFL has increased substantially since that benefit's creation in 2001. Consequently, active-duty personnel make up only 14 percent of the TRICARE Prime and Select populations; retirees and dependents make up almost 60 percent (TRICARE, 2017). Retirees and dependents under age 65 outnumber active-duty service members and dependents. Figure 2.4 provides a breakdown of the DoD beneficiary population by group.

VHA Enrollees

As of September 30, 2016, there were approximately 20 million veterans in the United States, with 8.3 million enrollees in the VA health

**Figure 2.4
DoD Health Beneficiaries, by
Category, FY 2017**

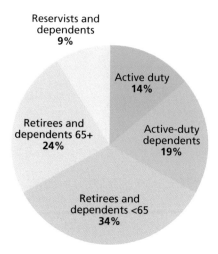

SOURCE: TRICARE, 2018b.

care system.[12] As described earlier, VA enrolls veterans according to priority group, with higher priority given to those with significant service-connected disabilities and low incomes. Figure 2.5 provides a breakdown of enrollment by priority group (priority groups 1–6 are considered high-priority). Of the 8.3 million VA enrollees on that date, only 6 million used VA health care in FY 2016.

Figure 2.5
VHA Enrollees, by Priority Group (millions)

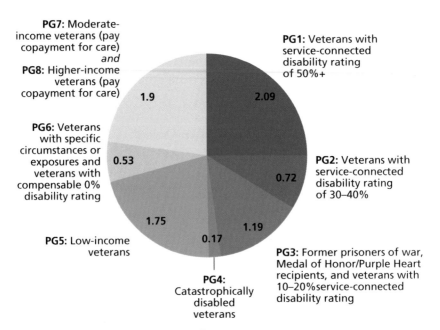

SOURCES: Huang et al., 2018; Panagala, 2016.
NOTE: PG = priority group.

<hr />

[12] The number of VA enrollees in Figure 2.5 differs from the number reported earlier in this report because the figure shows the total number of enrollees on a specific date. For the purposes of its enrollee survey, VA calculates the total number of enrollees on a given date, which differs from the total number enrolled over the course of the fiscal year.

Comparison of Populations

As noted, the MHS and VHA systems serve two distinct but overlapping populations. While the total population sizes seem relatively comparable (9.4 million in TRICARE and 8.3 million in VHA), it is important to understand the differences between TRICARE beneficiaries and VA enrollees in terms of relevant demographic characteristics, particularly age, since age is a critical factor in determining the potential health care needs and demand for services.

As shown in Table 2.2, a much larger proportion of the VA enrollee population is over age 65 (48 percent) than the TRICARE beneficiary population (24 percent), who for the most part enroll in Medicare and use TFL instead of the options relevant to the civilian provider network. On the other end of the age range, there are no VA enrollees under age 18, while children make up 21 percent of the TRICARE beneficiary population. These significant age differences are important when considering the requirements for an integrated purchased care network, which would need to ensure the availability of care for the combined population of VA enrollees and TRICARE

Table 2.2
Size of Populations, by Age Group

Age Group (years)	TRICARE Beneficiaries		VA Enrollees[b]	
	Number	%	Number	%
Birth–17	1,952,089	20.7%	0	0%
18–44	3,190,750	33.9%	1,717,194	20.6%
45–64	2,029,395	21.6%	2,585,948	31.0%
65+[a]	2,243,909	23.8%	4,042,286	48.4%
Total	9,416,143	100.0%	8,345,428	100%

[a] Most, but not all, of the 2.2 million DoD beneficiaries over age 65 are enrolled in Medicare and do not receive health care from TRICARE network providers. A small proportion are enrolled in TRICARE Prime, however.

[b] The size and breakdown of the VHA enrollees come from the 2017 VHA survey of enrollees (Huang et al., 2018); the data reflect a point-in-time overall population size, which may vary by month. The size and breakdown of DoD beneficiaries comes from the FY 2017 TRICARE report to Congress, which uses an end of fiscal year total.

beneficiaries. There are other differences between the two populations (e.g., where they live, their health care needs) that are critical to understand because they relate to how to design and manage an integrated purchased care network. For example, Figures 2.1 and 2.2 show that TRICARE beneficiaries tend to be clustered near military installations in urban areas, while VA enrollees are more likely to live in rural areas.

VA patients tend to be sicker overall than the general population. For example, VA patients are more likely to have cancer, diabetes, hypertension, asthma, and mental health conditions than nonveterans, even when accounting for differences in age and sex between veterans and nonveterans (Eibner et al., 2015). There are few direct comparisons of the health care needs of VA enrollees and TRICARE beneficiaries, but one study compared the health needs of VA patients under age 35 and service members under age 35. In that study, VA patients were more likely to have mental health conditions than similarly aged service members, while service members were more likely to have musculoskeletal conditions (Eibner et al., 2015).

About 1.5 million individuals are both enrolled in VA health care and have TRICARE coverage, a result of their eligibility for VA health care as veterans and their TRICARE eligibility as DoD retirees. This dual-eligible population accounts for 20 percent of the VA enrollee population and 16 percent of the DoD TRICARE beneficiary population (see Figure 2.6).

However, many dual-eligible individuals are age 65 or over and would likely not be accessing the TRICARE provider network; most are enrolled in TFL and receive care from Medicare providers.

Individuals who are both TRICARE beneficiaries and VA enrollees are likely different from those with only one form of coverage. For example, a survey of VA enrollees found that enrollees in priority groups 1–3 were more likely than those in lower-priority groups to have TRICARE coverage (one-third had TRICARE coverage, compared with less than 10 percent of those in higher-priority groups) (Huang et al., 2018).

Figure 2.6
Individuals Who Are Both TRICARE Beneficiaries and VA Enrollees

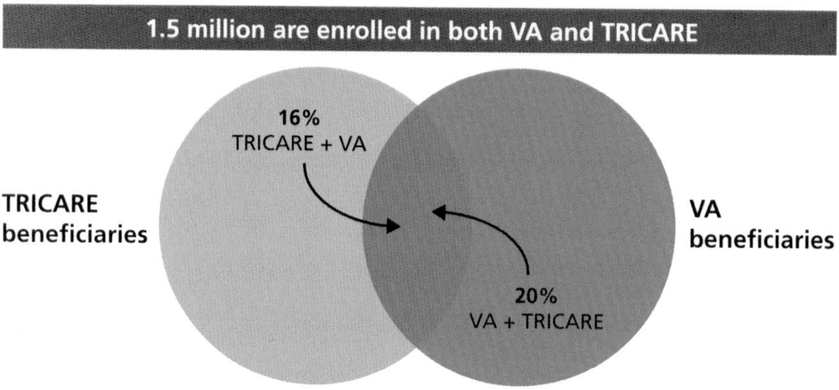

1.5 million are enrolled in both VA and TRICARE

16%
TRICARE + VA

TRICARE
beneficiaries

VA
beneficiaries

20%
VA + TRICARE

SOURCE: DoD data from an FY 2015 data match; VA data from Huang et al., 2018.

Summary

Through its TRICARE program, the MHS covers 9.4 million eligible beneficiaries, including active-duty service members, reserve service members, retired military personnel, and their dependents through services delivered in military-owned treatment facilities and purchased from the private sector. Both the MHS and the VA health care system offer this mix of direct and purchased care, with purchased care delivered through networks established and managed by contractors known as TPAs.

There are different eligibility requirements for the different TRICARE programs. And although TRICARE beneficiaries can access any private, community-based provider they choose, whether TRICARE will pay for the services varies based on the plan in which the patient is enrolled and whether the provider is part of the TRICARE network.

Through VHA, VA operates the largest integrated health care organization in the United States, with eligibility for care based on length of service, having a service-connected health condition, income, and other factors. Most veterans who are enrolled in VA health care have other sources of health coverage (e.g., Medicare, TRICARE, employer-sponsored insurance) and use VA to meet, on average, 30 percent of their health care needs.

The MHS and VHA systems serve two different but overlapping populations. While the total population sizes seem relatively comparable (9.4 million in TRICARE and 8.3 million in VHA), there are significant demographic differences between enrollees, particularly in terms of age—a critical factor in determining potential health care needs and demand for services.

Not all VHA-enrolled veterans are eligible to receive care in the community. If VA is unable to provide specific required health care services, it authorizes the purchase of that care from the private sector through one of its existing contract mechanisms. Only that episode of care is then authorized to be purchased in the private sector. VHA enrollees who are eligible for purchased care have a choice with respect to whom they seek care from in the community; they must work with the TPA or with VHA to ensure that the provider is eligible to receive payments from VHA. The recently passed VA MISSION Act requires VA establish new eligibility criteria for purchased care that consider patient preference and the quality of care available from a veteran's assigned VA facility.

CHAPTER THREE

DoD and VA Use of Purchased Care and Overview of Existing Purchased Care Provider Networks

As noted in the previous chapter, while both DoD and VA purchase care from the private sector, the departments have different missions and serve different, though overlapping, populations. We analyzed data provided by the two departments to identify differences in the type of care that DoD and VA purchase from the community. We also compared the networks of community providers contracted by DoD and VA.

Differences in Purchased Care Use

We requested data from the TRICARE Health Plan and the VA Office of Community Care on purchased care utilization for their covered populations. We analyzed the aggregate data provided by DoD and VA on the total number of purchased care visits (TRICARE) and authorizations (VA) in FY 2017. The TRICARE data included total counts of outpatient visits and inpatient admissions by type of care (e.g., primary care, specialty care) and patient characteristics (age, gender). The VA data included total counts of authorizations for purchased care, by category of care (e.g., specialty or type) and patient characteristics (age, gender). To compare TRICARE and VA purchased care utilization, we grouped VA categories of care to match TRICARE types of care: inpatient, surgery, emergency care, primary care, oncology, obstetrics/ gynecology (OB/GYN), cardiology, mental health care, and other.

The age and gender of patients receiving purchased care through TRICARE and VA differed considerably. Men accounted for the majority (87 percent in FY 2017) of VA purchased care authorizations, while women accounted for more than half (57 percent) of TRICARE purchased care visits (Figure 3.1). Patients under age 25 accounted for

Figure 3.1
DoD and VA Purchased Care Utilization, by Age and Gender, 2017

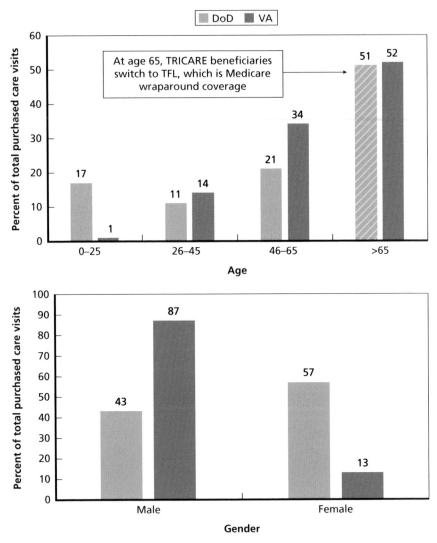

SOURCE: FY 2017 DoD and VA data.

17 percent of TRICARE purchased care visits in 2017 but only 1 percent of VA purchased care. For both TRICARE and VA, individuals over age 65 accounted for half of all purchased care visits or authorizations in FY 2017. However, it is important to recall that Medicare-eligible TRICARE beneficiaries who are enrolled in TFL receive care through Medicare, not the TRICARE network.[1] Figure 3.2 illustrates the differences between DoD and VA in purchased care use by age group when TFL beneficiaries are excluded.

Type of Health Care Purchased

TRICARE and VA purchase different types of care, reflecting differences in health needs between their covered populations and the role of purchased care in each system. The majority of our interviewees commented that differences in health care needs between TRICARE

Figure 3.2
DoD (excluding TFL) and VA Purchased Care Utilization, by Age, 2017

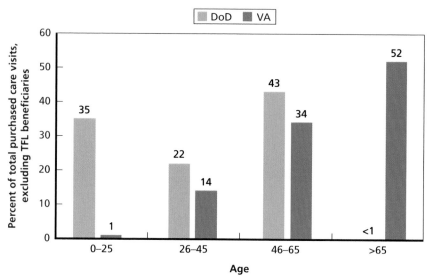

SOURCE: FY 2017 DoD and VA data.

---

[1] Some of the TFL beneficiaries' Medicare providers may also be in the TRICARE network; however, their participation in the network is not relevant for DoD reimbursement.

beneficiaries and VA enrollees are reflected in the type of care that the two health systems purchase from the private sector. We examined differences in purchased care use between the departments across nine types of care (inpatient, surgery, emergency care, primary care, oncology, OB/GYN, cardiology, and mental health care) as a proportion of all purchased care visits/admissions (TRICARE) or authorizations (VA).[2] Because TRICARE beneficiaries who are enrolled in TFL do not receive care from TRICARE network providers, we calculated TRICARE utilization two ways: including TFL beneficiaries (Figure 3.3) and excluding them (Figure 3.4). We focus here on the comparison between VA purchased care utilization and TRICARE

Figure 3.3
Utilization of VA and DoD Purchased Care, by Category of Care (including TFL), 2017

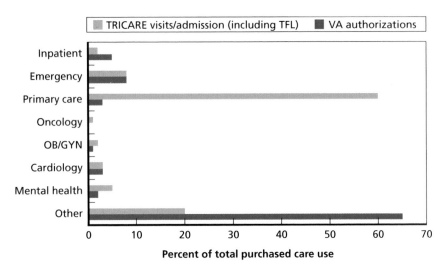

SOURCE: FY 2017 VA and DoD data.

---

[2]   VA authorizations included in the "other" category include specialty care services, such as endocrinology, gastroenterology, podiatry, neurology, dermatology, and ophthalmology. Utilization data for these specialties were not available from DoD in a disaggregated format, so we could not make comparisons across VA and DoD utilization patterns for these categories of care.

Figure 3.4
Utilization of VA and DoD Purchased Care, by Category of Care
(excluding TFL), 2017

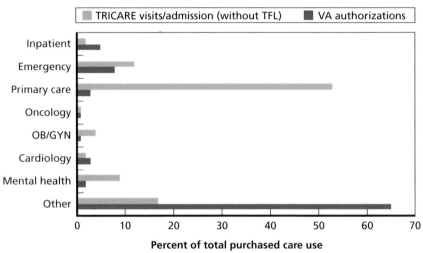

SOURCE: FY 2017 VA and DoD data.

utilization without TFL, as this comparison is most relevant for an integrated purchased care network.

Primary care makes up more than half (53 percent) of all purchased care visits for TRICARE but a very small proportion (3 percent) of VA purchased care authorizations. This is likely due to the differences in how and why DoD and VA purchase care. VA retains primary responsibility for patient care, referring patients to purchased care only for specific episodes of care, and, thus, almost all primary care is provided by VA providers in VA facilities. In contrast, TRICARE TPAs manage all care for some TRICARE beneficiaries (e.g., those enrolled in TRICARE Select), so primary care is provided through the TRICARE network rather than in MTFs.

Differences Between TRICARE and VA Purchased Care Provider Networks

To determine how similar or different the TRICARE and VA purchased care provider networks were, we analyzed individual provider-level data from DoD and VA for all providers in each network.[3] The provider data included provider name, office address (multiple records if more than one office location), and specialty. We chose to define geographic areas—specifically, counties—as the best available proxy for medical market area. We matched office zip code to county using the Centers for Disease Control and Prevention classification (CDC, 2014) and created a record for each unique provider-county combination; providers with offices in more than one county had multiple records, one for each county where they worked. Using the specialty information included in the files, we grouped providers into specialties as shown in Table 3.1. Some TRICARE providers had more than one specialty listed; in those cases, we selected the first specialty.

Figure 3.5 shows the overlap across the two networks by provider specialty group. Just under 30 percent of providers contract separately with both the TRICARE and VA networks. With the exception of pediatrics, this percentage varies only a little across specialty groups. The relatively few pediatrics specialists found in the VA network most likely either provide care for adults in addition to children, are included in a large multispecialty group, or provide care to newborn infants of VA-enrolled mothers.[4]

The modest overlap in the current networks is not surprising, given the population differences in the utilization of purchased care and differences in the types of care purchased from the private sector, as discussed earlier. Figure 3.6 shows the overlap in the two networks by county population density. The percentage of providers in both networks varies only a little by county type. A greater proportion of con-

---

[3]   The provider list from VA included all network providers contracted through either the Veterans Choice program or PC3. It did not include providers who contracted with VA through individual provider agreements.

[4]   VA covers care for newborns for the first seven days after birth for eligible women veterans who receive VA maternity care.

Table 3.1
Specialty Groups for Network Provider Analysis

Specialty Group	Examples of Specialties Included	TRICARE Network Providers (N = 655,107)	VA Network Providers (N = 510,664)
Adult primary care	General practice physician, family practitioner, general internist, primary care nurse practitioner, primary care physician assistant	217,950	131,683
Pediatrics	Pediatrician, pediatric subspecialist (including surgical subspecialist), pediatric nurse practitioner	42,868	5,263
OB/GYN	Obstetrician/gynecologist, midwife, OB/GYN nurse practitioner	25,712	16,208
Adult mental health	Psychiatrist, psychologist, social worker, behavioral medicine specialist, counselor, clinical social worker	86,108	46,682
Adult specialties	Medical subspecialist, surgical specialist, pathologist, anesthesiologist, nurse anesthetist, radiologist	191,693	237,966
Other	Chiropractor, podiatrist, optometrist, physical therapist	90,776	72,862

tracted providers in more rural areas contract only with VA, while a greater proportion in urban areas contract only with TRICARE.

As described in the previous chapter, the two beneficiary populations live in somewhat different locations (see Figures 2.1 and 2.2 in Chapter Two). TRICARE beneficiaries are more likely to live in urban areas, whereas more VA enrollees live in rural areas. Many of the largest cities have no MTF. In contrast, VA has large hospitals with a full range of specialty care in almost all urban areas of any size.

Figure 3.5
Nationwide Percentage of Providers in Both Networks, TRICARE Network Only, and VA Network Only, by Specialty Group

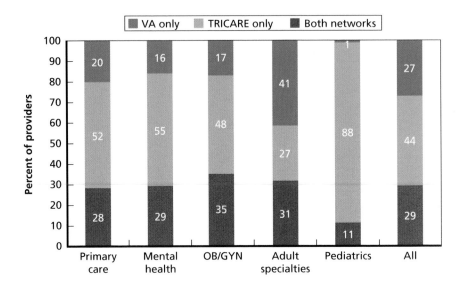

Summary

The age and gender of patients receiving purchased care through TRICARE and VA differed considerably. Men accounted for the majority (87 percent in FY 2017) of VA purchased care authorizations, while women accounted for more than half (57 percent) of TRICARE purchased care visits. Patients under age 25 accounted for 17 percent of TRICARE purchased care visits in 2017 but only 1 percent of VA purchased care. For both TRICARE and VA, individuals over age 65 accounted for half of all purchased care visits or authorizations in FY 2017. However, it is important to recall that Medicare-eligible TRICARE beneficiaries who are enrolled in TFL receive care through Medicare, not from the TRICARE network.

TRICARE and VA also purchase different types of care, reflecting differences in health needs between their covered populations and the role of purchased care in each system. We examined differences in

Figure 3.6
Nationwide Percentage of Providers in Both Networks, TRICARE Network Only, and VA Network Only, by County Type

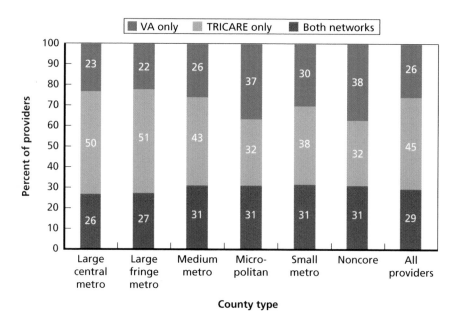

purchased care use across nine types of care, measured as a proportion of all purchased care visits/admissions (TRICARE) or authorizations (VA). We found that primary care makes up more than half (53 percent) of all purchased care visits for TRICARE but a very small proportion (3 percent) of VA purchased care authorizations, likely due to differences in how and why the two departments purchase care.

We also identified overlap across the two networks. Just under 30 percent of providers contract separately with both the TRICARE and VA networks, but this rate varied across provider specialty groups. When we assessed this overlap geographically, we found that a greater proportion of providers in rural areas contracted only with VA, while a greater proportion in urban areas contracted only with TRICARE. This distribution aligns with the distribution of their patients, with TRICARE beneficiaries more likely to live in urban areas and VA enrollees more likely to live in rural areas.

CHAPTER FOUR

Legal and Regulatory Authorities Underlying an Integrated Approach to Purchased Care for DoD and VA

In considering an integrated approach to purchased care for DoD and VA, including a single contract that would serve both departments, we started our feasibility assessment with an analysis of the legal and regulatory challenges and opportunities. To understand the legal and regulatory permissibility of integrating purchased care for DoD and VA, we examined existing legislative and regulatory authorities that govern how the departments furnish and purchase care. In this chapter, we first describe these authorities and then examine how these authorities address various dimensions of sharing or integration for the delivery of purchased care services.

Is Integrating Purchased Care Permissible Under Current Legislation and Regulations?

What Purchased Care Authorities Does DoD Currently Operate Under?

DoD has authority to purchase care for active-duty service members, reservists, dependents, and certain retirees. 10 U.S.C. 1073a states,

> Health care contracts shall be . . . to the offeror or offerors that will provide the best value to the United States to the maximum extent consistent with furnishing high-quality health care in a manner that protects the fiscal and other interests of the United States.

As described in prior chapters, DoD health care is offered to service members, dependents, and retirees through direct care provided in MTFs and through TRICARE, which offers are several plan options. These TRICARE options all allow beneficiaries to visit civilian health providers, to a greater or lesser degree depending on the program. DoD also has authority to enter into resource-sharing agreements with civilian health care providers, which could take a variety of forms, such as supplements to existing DoD direct care or purchased care, partnerships with academic medical centers, or other types of agreements. This resource sharing is allowed by statute if the agreement "would result in the delivery of health care in a more effective, efficient, or economical manner" (10 U.S.C. 1096; also see 32 C.F.R. 199.17[h]). These terms can apply to contracts for medical care for spouses and children (10 U.S.C. 1079); health benefits for certain service members, former service members, and their dependents (10 U.S.C. 1079); and alternative delivery methods for health care for retirees, dependents, and survivors, including HMOs, PPOs, individual providers, and consortia of providers (10 U.S.C. 1097).

What Purchased Care Authorities Does VA Currently Operate Under?

Until the signing of the VA MISSION Act in June 2018, VA operated under a fragmented set of statutory authorities for purchased care that evolved over several decades (Greenberg et al., 2015). These authorities exist (or existed) primarily in Title 38 of the U.S. Code, the federal statutes governing VA. Under these statutes, VA had the authority to purchase care on a "fee basis" for single instances or episodes of care when "economical" services were not available from VA due to "geographical inaccessibility" or when VA facilities were not capable of "furnishing the care or services required" (38 U.S.C. 1703). Title 38 also gave VA the authority to purchase emergency care when there was reasonable expectation that delay in care "would have been hazardous to life or health" (38 U.S.C. 1725, 1728). A parallel set of authorities in Title 38 allowed for provider sharing when "sharing of medical facilities, equipment, and information" with any provider would be "in the best interest of the prevailing standards" of VA. In practice, this authority has been used to facilitate VA's entrance into long-term contracts for purchasing specific types of care or services from medical schools, health care facilities, and research centers (38 U.S.C. 8151–8158). In the 2014 Veterans Choice Act, Congress gave VA the authority to purchase care when a veteran is unable to schedule an appointment within certain VA "wait-time goals," resides more than 40 miles from a VA medical facility (less, under certain conditions), must travel by air or water, or faces "unusual or excessive" "geographic challenges" to reach a VA medical facility.[1] VA implemented this Choice Act authority by modifying its existing PC3 contracts to purchase care for veterans in significant quantities from its two large health services contractors (Health Net and Tri-West).

The VA MISSION Act, signed on June 6, 2018, consolidated and altered much of this structure (Pub. L. 115-182, 2018). As of this writing, the act's new authorities were to be implemented over the following year, with veterans receiving care under the Choice Act or other purchased care authorities grandfathered in as beneficiaries of the new VA MISSION Act programs.[2] Section 101 of the VA MISSION Act establishes a "program to furnish hospital care, medical services, and extended care services to covered veterans through health care providers." The act specifically includes DoD in its list of health care providers with which VA may contracts.

The VA MISSION Act replaced some of the earlier statutory language giving VA authority to contract for services with two new statutory sections. The first described a "tiered network" to be developed by VA for the purchase of care:

(g) TIERED NETWORK.—

(1) To promote the provision of high-quality and high-value hospital care, medical services, and extended care services under this

---

[1] 38 U.S.C. 1701 note, as codified by Pub. L. 113-146, 2014, 128 Stat. 1754, 1757.

[2] The VA MISSION Act was not to take effect until at least a year after signing, either when the VA Secretary submitted a report required under the Choice Act or when the VA Secretary promulgated new regulations relating to the purchase of care when or where VA facilities were found to be substandard, whichever occurred later.

section, the Secretary may develop a tiered provider network of eligible providers based on criteria established by the Secretary for purposes of this section.

(2) In developing a tiered provider network of eligible providers under paragraph (1), the Secretary shall not prioritize providers in a tier over providers in any other tier in a manner that limits the choice of a covered veteran in selecting a health care provider specified in subsection (c) for receipt of hospital care, medical services, or extended care services under this section. (38 U.S.C. 1703(g), as amended by Pub. L. 115-182)

The second new purchased care authority in the VA MISSION Act described the mechanics of contracting more specifically:

(h) CONTRACTS TO ESTABLISH NETWORKS OF HEALTH CARE PROVIDERS.—

(1) The Secretary shall enter into consolidated, competitively bid contracts to establish networks of health care providers specified in paragraphs (1) and (5) of subsection (c) for purposes of providing sufficient access to hospital care, medical services, or extended care services under this section.

(2)(A) The Secretary shall, to the extent practicable, ensure that covered veterans are able to make their own appointments using advanced technology.

(B) To the extent practicable, the Secretary shall be responsible for the scheduling of appointments for hospital care, medical services, and extended care services under this section. (38 U.S.C. 1703(h), as amended by Pub. L. 115-182)

Notably, the VA MISSION Act's payment provision gives VA authority to "incorporate, to the extent practicable, the use of value-based reimbursement models to promote the provision of high-quality care." This is significant because of the congressional direction to DoD to use value-based reimbursement models for TRICARE (see, e.g., Pub. L. 114-328, 2016, Sec. 705). For the first time, VA may have explicit statutory authority to use value-base reimbursement for its contracting, potentially aligning the VA and DoD purchased care business models.

To What Extent Do DoD and VA Authorities Enable Each to Purchase Care from or Through Another Federal Agency (other than DoD or VA) or That Agency's Contracts?

Each department's authorities and appropriations (see Table 4.1) for purchased care generally allow it to purchase care for its beneficiaries, subject to various restrictions. DoD's statutory authorities refer to TRI-CARE as a specific program and contract. VA's authorities (as revised by the VA MISSION Act) refer to the "Veterans Community Care Program" and direct VA toward "a program to furnish hospital care, medical services, and extended care services to covered veterans" through one of several health care providers, including DoD and its contrac-

Table 4.1
Assessment of Existing Authorities to Purchase Care

Question	Answer
Can DoD or VA use the other's contract (Veterans Choice or TRICARE) to purchase care for its beneficiaries?	Yes, under existing authorities to purchase care for their beneficiaries, existing appropriations for that care, and government-wide authorities to purchase goods or services through other agencies. However, DoD and VA would need strict controls in place to ensure that their appropriations went only to their beneficiaries, and that these beneficiaries were reimbursed for all direct and indirect costs, in the absence of some new Joint Incentive Fund or other joint appropriation.
Do current "resource-sharing" statutes (e.g., 38 U.S.C. 8111) enable joint contracting?	Maybe, although congressional staff expressed an opinion that these authorities were meant for narrower pilot programs and that members of Congress would likely be skeptical of large-scale resource sharing without new authority.
Do current appropriations support a joint contract for DoD and VA?	No, because current appropriations language specifically mentions the contractual programs used by DoD and VA. Future appropriations statutes would need to be adjusted to incorporate the new joint contract structure and give them flexibility to purchase care through means other than their own current contracts.

tors. DoD appropriations contain one large account for the Defense Health Program, including a portion for TRICARE; VA's appropriations come in five separate accounts, one of which is specifically for VA community care. This difference, along with DoD authority to move funds within the Defense Health Program account (10 U.S.C. 1100), enables DoD to reprogram money within its appropriations account structure more easily than VA.

The VA MISSION Act also contains specific language making DoD a health care provider for the purposes of VA purchased care. Under these authorities and appropriations, each department could likely purchase care for its beneficiaries by adding the other or its providers to its current contracts as subcontractors. Each department can also use its current appropriations to pay for *its own* beneficiaries' care, if that care were purchased through the programs described in those appropriations. However, notwithstanding the resource-sharing authorities (e.g., 38 U.S.C. 8111), DoD and VA would likely need new statutory authority for a joint, integrated contract and would also likely need different appropriations language to purchase care through a joint, integrated contract. Such a joint contract would also need to be carefully constructed to ensure that each agency paid for direct and indirect costs associated with its beneficiaries only.

Federal government contracts are regulated by a combination of statute and policy. The major statutory provisions for civilian agencies are contained in Title 41 of the U.S. Code, while the major statutory provisions for DoD contracts are contained in Title 10. In general, these statutory rules mirror each other (such as the Competition in Contracting Act of 1984, which exists in substantially similar form in both Title 10 and Title 41).[3]

There are meaningful differences between the civilian and DoD procurement statutes, however, including differences regarding competitive selection procedures and bid protests and requirements for reporting to Congress. Below the level of statute, federal government contracts are governed by the FAR. This voluminous regulation is codified in Title 48 of the Code of Federal Regulations and is managed by

---

[3] See 41 U.S.C. 253 and 10 U.S.C. 2304.

a triagency council led by DoD, the National Aeronautics and Space Administration (NASA), and the General Services Administration. The FAR sets rules applicable to all government contracts. However, each agency has its own acquisition supplement: DFARS for DoD and VAAR for VA. These DoD and VA acquisition regulations are reflected in the TRICARE and VA community care contracts, respectively, with many regulatory requirements incorporated into contractual clauses either in full text or by reference. Depending on the structure of a joint contract, and which entity it falls under, any differences between the Title 10 and 41 statutory requirements, as well as the DFARS and VAAR requirements, would need to be reconciled. These differences include treatment of organizational conflicts of interest, rules for the treatment of costs, and the application of certain agency-unique statutes, such as VA's statutory mandate to contract with veteran-owned businesses (38 U.S.C. 8127).

What Resource-Sharing or Joint Contracting Authorities Currently Exist for DoD and VA?

Historically, DoD and VA have partnered in several areas in treating service members and veterans. These efforts have included centers focused on severely wounded, ill, or injured veterans, such as VA's polytrauma centers or the James A. Lovell Federal Health Care Center in North Chicago, established as a pilot program in 2010. According to a 2015 DHA briefing, at that time, 61 VA medical facilities had partnered with 97 MTFs, "for a total of 187 direct sharing agreements in delivery of 117 unique services."[4] These partnerships rest on a foundation of legal authority found throughout Titles 10 and 38 of the U.S. Code. The most significant of these resource-sharing authorities are as follows:

- 38 U.S.C. 8111 provides broad authority for DoD and VA to share health care resources, directing the two departments to "enter into agreements and contracts for the mutually benefi-

---

[4] According to an August 10, 2015, briefing, "DoD VA Health Care Collaboration," provided to RAND for this study.

cial coordination, use, or exchange of use of the VA and DoD health care resources with the goal of improving the access to, and quality and cost effectiveness of, the health care provided by VHA and the MHS to the beneficiaries of both departments."

- 10 U.S.C. 1104 mirrors 38 U.S.C. 8111, authorizing the Secretary of Defense to share departmental health care resources with VA health care resources in accordance with 38 U.S.C. 8111, or under 31 U.S.C. 1535, the federal Economy Act statute for purchasing goods or services through other agencies' contracts. Notably, this authority also authorizes the Secretary of Defense to reimburse VA for health care services. Furthermore, in times of war or national emergency (as was the case at the time of this writing), 10 U.S.C. 1104 also authorizes DoD to use VA health care services for active-duty personnel under VA authority for wartime resource sharing (38 U.S.C. 8111A).

- 38 U.S.C. 8111 and the Joint Incentive Fund, are intended "to provide seed money and incentives for innovative DoD/VA joint sharing initiatives to recapture purchased care, improve quality and drive cost savings at facilities," according to DHA (MHS, undated[e]). The Joint Incentive Fund was established by the National Defense Authorization Act for FY 2003 (Pub. L. 107-314, 2002), which required DoD and VA to contribute $15 million to the fund annually. In FY 2015, DoD and VA jointly funded 66 projects through the Joint Incentive Fund.

DoD Instruction 6010.23 addresses DoD and VA health care resource sharing under the two statutory authorities. The policy states,

> The DoD and VA shall enter into direct care sharing agreements and contracts for the mutually beneficial coordination, use, and exchange of health care resources of their departments. The goal of sharing agreements is to improve access to, and quality, efficiency, and effectiveness of the health care provided by the MHS and VHA to their respective beneficiaries. (U.S. Department of Defense Instruction 6010.23, 2013, p. 2)

The instruction also states that VA health care facilities may directly enter into network provider agreements with MCSCs.[5] Under these agreements, the VA facility is the authorized participating provider, the MCSC reimburses the VA facility, and the referral of eligible DoD beneficiaries to VA facilities is managed by the MCSC (U.S. Department of Defense Instruction 6010.23, 2013, p. 11).

Congressional staff described these authorities as less about sharing, *per se*, and more about treating each other's patients and seeking reimbursement later. Congressional staff also said that these authorities were intended to provide a legal basis for pilot programs or tests, not for wide-scale integration of DoD and VA's purchased care networks. Use of these authorities for large-scale network sharing may trigger congressional scrutiny. Current usage is reportedly small (about $100 million purchased by each department from the other annually).

To What Extent Do DoD and VA Authorities Enable Each to Provide Care to the Other's Beneficiaries Without Necessarily Purchasing Such Care?

Neither DoD nor VA has general authority to provide care to the other's beneficiaries. DoD has some limited authority to send active service members to VA for health care in times of war or national emergency, as well as to reimburse VA for this care (10 U.S.C. 1104; 38 U.S.C. 8111A). DoD also has authority under the VA MISSION Act to serve as a health care provider as part of the VA Community Care Program, although DoD would ostensibly be reimbursed for this care by VA. VA's authority in this sphere enables it to purchase care to support active-duty personnel for whom it must provide care. However, VA does not have any general authority to provide care to the active or reserve population, except to those who have completed a term of service and have been discharged by DoD such that they have earned VA care and benefits. VA also lacks authority to provide care for the dependents of active and reserve personnel, save for its narrow authorities regarding caregivers. Conversely, DoD lacks statutory authority to

---

[5] MCSCs are responsible for administering TRICARE in each region.

care for veterans beyond their discharge,[6] except for DoD retirees who may continue to obtain care at an MTF or via TRICARE, or for service members within their first six months after discharge, who retain TRICARE eligibility (TRICARE, undated[b]).

Do Any Government-Wide Authorities Enable the Purchase of Care Through a Joint Contract?

According to Volume 11A of the DoD Financial Management Regulation, para 030102 (2012),

> The Economy Act (31 U.S.C. 1535) provides the authority for federal agencies to order goods and services from major organizations within the same agency or other federal agencies and to pay the actual costs of those goods and services.

The regulation authorizes agencies to contract with other agencies for goods or services, if they're available, if it is in the best interests of the government, if the agency is able to get or contract for the goods or services, and if the goods or services cannot be provided as cheaply or conveniently by a commercial enterprise (31 U.S.C. 1535–1536). This authority would enable DoD or VA to purchase care through another agency's contract. In accordance with 10 U.S.C. 2205, "reimbursements made to DoD appropriations under 31 U.S.C. 1535 and 1536 for services rendered or supplies furnished, may be credited to the appropriation or fund of the activity performing the reimbursable work" (DoD Financial Management Regulation, Vol. 11A, para. 030104C, 2012). Details about these interagency acquisitions are provided in the FAR, Subpart 17.5, "Interagency Acquisitions." There are some important limitations on the use of the Economy Act for acquisitions due to historical abuses, such as the rule that orders under the act "may not be used by an agency to circumvent conditions and limitations imposed on the use of funds, including extending the period of availability of

---

[6]   The exception to this rule is DoD's authority to provide TRICARE coverage to veterans beyond their discharge, including six months of coverage for all discharged service members, or longer coverage for those who purchase TRICARE under COBRA rules. See TRICARE, undated(a), undated(b).

the cited funds" (DoD Financial Management Regulation, Vol. 11A, para. 030105, 2012). In addition, it does not appear that a comparable contract has been procured under the Economy Act that matches the size, scope, or complexity of a joint DoD-VA purchased care contract, nor that any agency has in place the type of reciprocal reimbursement arrangements needed for this type of contract.

What Legal Gaps or Barriers Would Impede DoD or VA from Purchasing Care Through a Joint Contract?

Three types of legal obstacles would impede DoD and VA from pursuing a joint contract to purchase care for their respective beneficiaries. The first of these are differences in authorities, which describe each department's program (TRICARE and VA Community Care) and would need to be amended by Congress to enable the purchase of care through some new joint contract or program.

The second set of legal barriers exist within the appropriations structures for each department. DoD could likely use its TRICARE appropriations to purchase care through a joint contract, given that these funds all fall within the broad scope of the Defense Health Program appropriation, and DoD has some legal authority to reprogram funds (subject to congressional notice and consent requirements). However, VA may need more permissive appropriations language than it has now for its Community Care account or a separate appropriation for the joint contract, such as more funds for the DoD-VA Joint Incentive Fund. Relatedly, each department's portion of the contract would have to be carefully managed to conform to the eligibility requirements in each department's statute, which differ substantially and would need to be managed at each step of the process—from appointments scheduling through reimbursement and insurance billing.

Third, beneath the level of these legal barriers, there are also myriad policy, regulatory and practical barriers that would need to be addressed, from rewriting various DoD and VA policy documents to negotiating reimbursement mechanisms and cost allocation formulas for the joint contract's direct and indirect costs.

Different Eligibility Requirements in Statute

As noted in Chapter Two, there are eligibility differences between the DoD and VA programs. These eligibility differences matter to the extent that each department's authorities and appropriations may only, by law, be used to provide care for that department's eligible beneficiaries. DoD funds cannot pay for veterans' health care (unless those veterans are also DoD-eligible), and VA funds cannot pay for military dependents' health care (unless those dependents fall under VA's relatively narrow authorities for caregivers). This creates a statutory barrier to the integration of the two systems without legislative change. To function under existing authorities and appropriations, such a system would need to carefully separate the authorities and appropriations for each population and scrupulously account for costs (including direct and indirect costs, such as overhead) to ensure that department appropriations were being used for their statutory purposes.

Differences in Appropriations Processes

Both department's appropriations generally allow for their use to purchase care for its respective beneficiaries. There appear to be no limitations in DoD or VA appropriations that would preclude purchasing care for their respective beneficiaries through another contract vehicle or a joint contract vehicle, except to the extent that the current appropriations laws for FYs 2018 and 2019 refer to the TRICARE and Veterans Choice programs by name and would likely need to be amended if these appropriations were to go to some other contractual program.

On a more strategic level, DoD and VA have different mechanisms for forecasting, requesting, and allocating their appropriations. DoD and VA each use different systems to predict future health care demand and calculate the level of resources necessary to meet that demand. DoD's system exists both at the Office of the Secretary of Defense (OSD) level and the level of the services, which until FY 2019 maintained a significant portion of the DoD health care system (Pub. L. 115-232, Sec. 711–712). VA (including both VA Central Office and VHA leadership) uses a different forecasting model to determine future demand, as well as the resources necessary to meet that demand. Setting aside potential critiques of these models, they differ in their methodologies, data sources, populations considered, cost models, and outputs.

Each department then does something different with its outputs, based on its organizational and congressional appropriations structure. DoD estimates costs and budgets on a five-year cycle through a mechanism called the Planning, Programming, Budgeting, and Execution (PPBE) process. The PPBE includes plans from OSD for DoD-wide funding, as well as plans from each of the services. Although DoD plans five years in advance for its funding, it submits annual appropriations requests to Congress and receives annual appropriations from Congress for its operations (notwithstanding certain appropriations for multiyear items, such as construction or the acquisition of major weapon systems).

VA, by contrast, is beginning to implement its own version of the DoD PPBE process to plan appropriations over five-year cycles, but this effort is not yet as mature as the DoD PPBE process. However, the main difference is in the "advance appropriations" system that applies to VA health care by law (38 U.S.C. 117). Each year, the department requests both its appropriation for the coming year and an advance appropriation for the following fiscal year. VA requests (and receives) these appropriations on a rolling basis and reconciles the difference between the advance appropriation and the current appropriation each year, as necessary (see Tollestrup, 2015). VA's advanced appropriation system insulates it from turbulence associated with congressional failures to timely reach agreements on budget and spending legislation, as well as from potential legal risk under the Anti-Deficiency Act, which makes it unlawful for federal agencies to incur obligations without appropriated funds (31 U.S.C. 1341). This differentiates VA health funding from DoD health funding, as the latter does not get the benefit of advance appropriations.

Congress differs in the types of appropriations that it gives to each department as well. Historically, Congress has appropriated a sum of funds for the Defense Health Program, including a specific amount within that appropriation for the TRICARE program. The level of generality for this appropriation enables some flexibility at the department level to move funds around within the overall Defense Health Program, or within the MTF or purchased care components of that program, within the bounds of DoD's reprogramming authorities.[7] By contrast, VA requests and receives appropriations in several separate accounts for its health care system. Until 2014, Congress divided its VA health care appropriations into four accounts: (1) medical services, (2) medical support and compliance, (3) medical facilities, and (4) medical and prosthetic research. In 2014, with the passage of the Veterans Choice Act, Congress began to appropriate funds for VA health care in a fifth account, which originally carried the name of the Veterans Choice program and is now known as VA Community Care. VA's appropriations structure limits the department's ability to move funds within the VA health care system and requires congressional consent to move funds in excess of 1 percent of the amounts appropriated (see Pub. L. 115-244, 2018, Sec. 202, Title II, Div. C).

There are some added complexities within the systems as well. DoD accrues funds to pay for the future health care of its retirees (and their dependents) in the DoD MERHCF. These funds are accrued each year and managed by a complex actuarial system; they are then used to pay the TRICARE costs of Medicare-eligible DoD retirees and their dependents, who are generally over the age of 65 (DoD, Office of the Actuary, 2016). Although this segment accounts for only one-quarter of the DoD beneficiary population, it is a costly one, so this accrual mechanism plays an important role in financing the overall Defense Health Program. There are no such mechanisms on the VA side to accrue funds as veterans age or as disability compensation is awarded. On the VA side, there are numerous complexities driven by the interaction between the VA health care system and the other health care options available to veterans, as well as the synergistic interaction among disability compensation, VA priority group status, and VA

---

[7] See, for example, 10 U.S.C. 126, 10 U.S.C. 2214, and Congressional Research Service, 2013. See also 10 U.S.C. 1100 (on giving DoD authority to move funds within the Defense Health Program account).

health care utilization. These complexities make it difficult to forecast demand with great precision, especially as new programs for VA care come into being, such as the Veterans Choice (now VA Community Care) program, that substantially expand access or change the nature of care. And, importantly, VA does not have legal authority to act as a supplement to Medicare or employer-provided insurance, nor to bill Medicare for services provided to Medicare-eligible veterans, making VA the primary payer for nearly all of its patients. Consequently, a joint contract would end up operating on substantially different financial terms for DoD beneficiaries (particularly DoD retirees and their family members who are Medicare-eligible) than for VA beneficiaries.

Summary

DoD and VA currently have authorities to purchase care for their beneficiaries, which they use to operate the current TRICARE and Veterans Choice contracting programs. These purchased care authorities are broad and would likely allow DoD or VA to purchase care through the other's contract—or from another agency's direct care facilities. Federal statute also contains authority for DoD and VA to share resources "with the goal of improving the access to, and quality and cost effectiveness of, the health care provided . . . to the beneficiaries of both Departments" (38 U.S.C. 8111), and Congress has given DoD and VA special authorities and appropriations mechanisms for small-scale pilots aimed at demonstrating the value and efficacy of joint DoD-VA health care. However, current authorities and appropriations would need to be amended to provide for a joint, integrated contracting approach to purchased care.

The broad purchased care authorities for each department would probably provide legal authority for participating in an integrated contract, but it is unclear whether the narrower resource-sharing authorities would do so, given their history and the opinions of congressional staff involved in the oversight of these authorities. Furthermore, current appropriations language limits the extent to which each department can purchase anything outside of the existing contractual programs.

Future contracting approaches, including a joint contracting approach, would need new language in future appropriations bills that directs funds to those new contracting programs instead of the legacy language tied to TRICARE or VA Community Care (formerly Choice). Given differences in budgeting and financial oversight, an increase in costs to VA for purchasing care may have an impact on other budget areas within VHA. Additional analyses will be needed to determine whether pursuing a joint contract would lead to increased costs that could impinge on resources for other VHA functions.

CHAPTER FIVE

Barriers with Respect to Operational Execution of an Integrated Purchased Care Approach

This chapter provides an overview of how DoD and VA execute their purchased care functions. This analysis is based on our review of TRI-CARE contracts, Veterans Choice contracts, VA PC3 contracts, and VA's RFP for its Community Care Network. We supplemented this review with interviews with representatives from current and former TRICARE and VA TPAs and benefits consulting firms in the private sector who were familiar with the operations of TPAs for employers.

We describe how DoD and VA define the roles of TPAs, how they administer their contracts, and how they incorporate industry standards for purchasing care. We also discuss how the departments compare and contrast across these dimensions to highlight the potential barriers and facilitators to an integrated approach.

Contracting Processes and Relationship with TPAs

In the private sector, the main role of a TPA is to take on administrative and other tasks for payers. In many instances, TPAs are themselves also payers; large health insurance firms have their own health plans and administer large, self-insured employer health plans. TPAs can also be organizations that specialize in administrative, behind-the-scenes processes, such as claims adjudication. TPAs perform a variety of functions for payers (primarily employers) that can be sorted into two broad categories. The first category is purely providing administrative services related to enrollment, claims adjudication, customer service, and maintaining a network of providers. The second is a set of additional services, such as providing recommendations on benefit design, utilization management services, population health monitoring and care or disease management services. The various roles of a TPA are summarized in Table 5.1.

Roles of TRICARE and VA TPAs

Both DoD and VA contract with TPAs to purchase care from the private sector. The role of the TRICARE TPAs (currently Health Net Federal Services and Humana Military) is to maintain a provider network, adjudicate claims, provide customer service, and conduct a variety of additional functions, such as quality reporting. The role of the TRICARE TPAs is similar to that in the private sector. The role of VA TPAs (currently Health Net Federal Services and TriWest) is to maintain a provider network, pay providers, provide customer service, and coordinate the sharing of medical record documentation between network providers and VA direct care facilities. The role of VA TPAs is much narrower than in the private sector or in TRICARE. One important difference from the private sector for both DoD and VA is that the departments determine the benefits furnished under each contract instead of relying on the TPAs to design the benefits. Cost sharing is set by legislation. This is in contrast to the private sector, in which TPAs play a much larger role in determining which services are covered and the associated cost sharing. One final key difference is that TPAs for both departments transmit medical records between the providers in the community and the DHA and VHA direct care systems for active-duty service members or veterans. There is no similar role for private-sector TPAs.

There are some differences in the roles of TPAs between the departments. The first is the scope of medical services that TPAs manage. The second difference is that TRICARE TPAs coordinate with MTFs to assign patients to MTFs or the community, while VA TPAs do not take on this function. The third is that TRICARE TPAs manage the full spectrum of utilization for beneficiaries (similar to an employer health plan), except for Prime enrollees managed by an MTF

Table 5.1
Key Roles of TPAs

Role	Definition
Maintain provider network	Establish payment contracts with individual providers or groups of providers to serve the enrolled population
Enrollment	Formally enroll an individual (or family) into a specific plan with a specific set of benefits[a]
Claim adjudication	Assess whether a service is covered under the plan's benefits, pays claim to provider
Customer service	Staff call centers, create informational websites, and handle appeals of service denials
Benefit design	Recommend medical services and prescription drugs to be covered and their associated cost-sharing arrangements (e.g., deductibles, copayments, coinsurance)
Utilization management	Create a set of tools used to ensure appropriate levels of service use that includes prior authorization (requiring TPA approval that the service is medically necessary before payment will be issued), step therapy (requiring that patients fail to respond to certain treatments before trying others that are usually more expensive), and quantity limits (limits on the quantity of service, such as the number of physical therapy visits per year)
Quality reporting	Report on quality metrics that usually derive from claims data and capture whether enrollees are receiving recommended care, their access to care, and their experiences with care with such tools as the commonly used HEDIS measure set
Population health management	Perform activities that include identifying when patients are not receiving recommended care and helping both the patient and providers resolve barriers to receiving recommended care
Care or disease management	Care management: Target high-cost enrollees or those at risk of using large amounts of medical care with extra services to ensure that they receive appropriate care; closely related to population health management
	Disease management: generally a lower level of service designed for a specific condition that includes education, tools for self-management of the disease, and other wellness activities, such as diet and exercise counseling, to mitigate risk factors

NOTE: HEDIS = Healthcare Effectiveness Data and Information Set, maintained by the National Committee for Quality Assurance. For more information, see NCQA, undated.

[a] Employers decide who is eligible for the health plan.

or other care received in an MTF. VA TPAs manage only small pieces of a veteran's overall health care utilization (usually single episodes of care). This fundamental difference limits the VA TPA's ability to predict demand for providers (amount of utilization), manage population health, and implement quality improvement measures. The fourth difference is that the TPAs fully process claims for DoD but not for VA. Currently, VA maintains control over claims processing.

Scope of Services

Under TRICARE contracts, the scope of medical services that the TPA manages differs depending on beneficiaries' plan type. For 2.8 million TRICARE beneficiaries, the TPA manages all medical care, following the model of most other TPA arrangements in the federal government and the private sector. It also processes civilian care claims and performs other, more limited functions for the remaining 6.6 million beneficiaries.

TRICARE Prime enrollees assigned to an MTF are required to have specific authorizations to receive care outside the MTF. In this regard, the MTFs act much like a staff-model HMO, in which purchased care is used only to supplement internal capabilities.[1] The TPA manages only the care that is referred to the private sector. The TPA also processes claims for the supplemental payments TRICARE makes for beneficiaries with other health insurance or TFL.

VA purchased care is similar to TRICARE Prime; VA providers manage most medical care for VA enrollees, and veterans receive outside care only under certain circumstances and only for an authorized episode of care. The TPA manages medical care associated with those authorized veterans' episodes of care, which means that the set of services required from community providers differs by VAMC and by veteran, and there are no standards across the country for which services are covered. Without standardized benefit structures, it is more difficult for TPAs to set up automatic claims adjudications for services.

---

[1]   A staff-model HMO is an organization that employs physicians and other medical staff and delivers medical care in return for a fixed amount of money per year. A common example is Kaiser Permanente.

Additionally, it can be difficult for the TPAs to maintain an ongoing provider network if they are unsure of the demand for services in specific geographic locations or from a given type of provider.

Direct Versus Community Care

TRICARE TPAs coordinate with MTFs to refer Prime enrollees to either an MTF or a civilian primary care provider and to direct referrals for enrollees in civilian care to an MTF, where available. MTFs have the "right of first refusal" for Prime enrollees referred for specialty care. Only if the MTF cannot provide the needed care can the care be referred out to the community.

TRICARE TPAs have a full window on the care utilization of Prime enrollees assigned to civilian primary care, so they can take on such functions as utilization or population health management for these Prime enrollees, similar to private-sector health insurers or TPAs. Under TRICARE Prime, MTFs have primary responsibility for utilization and population health management for enrollees assigned to an MTF primary care provider

In contrast, VA alone decides which services to refer out to the community. If the TPA does not have a role in managing where veterans receive care and which types of services are offered, it is more difficult to hold them responsible for utilization or population health management.

Quality Reporting

Both DoD and VA have directed their TPAs to use industry best practices to manage utilization. For example, both departments now ask TPAs to report on quality metrics used for commercial and Medicare Advantage plans: HEDIS and Consumer Assessment of Healthcare Providers and Systems (CAHPS) (HEDIS, 2018; AHRQ, 2018). Private-sector and Medicare Advantage health plans routinely collect the information needed to construct the measures from providers, from claims data, or from enrollees directly (for CAHPS) (Burns, 2017; NCQA, 2017). VA's new Community Care Network RFP listed several of the HEDIS measures that TPAs would track to identify high-performing providers, including measures related to diabetes care (e.g., whether blood sugar is controlled or whether the veteran has been monitored for kidney disease or received an eye exam) and appropriate screening for cancer.

The ability of VA TPAs to perform these functions remains limited because they do not see the majority of most veterans' care. This is an ongoing challenge for VA that would not be resolved with a joint contract. VA TPAs may not have visibility into care provided in a VAMC, nor would they have knowledge of care paid for by other payers. Many veterans have other sources of health care coverage, such as employer-sponsored insurance, Medicaid, or Medicare. In contrast, DoD TPAs receive data on MTF utilization and calculate quality measures for beneficiaries who receive care in the community. DoD TPAs do not calculate quality measures for active-duty personnel who receive care only from an MTF.

Claims Processing

Claims processes for DoD are fully electronic, and many are adjudicated automatically, a process assisted by a clear set of established rules for the covered services nationwide. DoD sends the TPAs advance payments to allow them to quickly pay providers and then audits those payments, rather than individual claim payment amounts. This process allows for a lower administrative overhead, since many claims are handled automatically. The TPA then focuses on performing utilization management functions, such as overseeing authorization of more-expensive or less-common procedures. In contrast, VA adjudicates and pays claims individually in-house. This is a manual process for each claim, though VA is establishing a new system to pay claims electronically according to common claims payment standards. In the current process, after care is delivered, VA TPAs pay the provider and then must wait for reimbursement from VA. VA adjudicates the amount, which in some cases is less than what the TPA paid the provider if VA does not approve of the services rendered. According to VA's Office of Community Care, moving forward with the new Community Care Network, VA will receive claims information electronically in an industry-standard format (EDI transaction) and will use a new IT solution to reimburse the TPA.[2] VA will no longer adjudicate individual claims and will require increased internal controls regarding claims payment from the TPAs.

Our interviews with current and former TPAs revealed differing opinions on whether DoD and VA would have to work out these underlying differences in administrative processes prior to pursuing a joint contract. Some interviewees thought that the process could be done in steps, such that the first contract would have a joint provider network and separate administrative processes that were harmonized over time. Others thought that VA would need to allow the TPA to have a greater role in claims processing and proactively managing networks (similar to TRICARE's current practices) for the joint contract to be effective. There was a belief that processes for providers should be harmonized to avoid confusion and dissatisfaction. Finally, some interviewees thought that piloting a joint contracting vehicle in particular areas would allow both departments to resolve many of these operational differences prior to rolling out a joint contract to entire regions.

Differences in Contract Terms

In this section, we review the contractual differences in the TPA contracts for VA and DoD as they relate to (1) network standards, (2) provider payment, (3) network participation requirements, and (4) reporting requirements and incentive structures. We include illustrative comparisons to private-sector and Medicare Advantage practices, where relevant.[3]

---

[2] Personal communication, September 2018.

[3] Under the Medicare Advantage program, commercial insurers contract with CMS to offer Medicare beneficiaries their Part A (hospital) and B (physician services) benefits and often include Part D (prescription drugs) in one package. Beneficiaries opt into the voluntary program and often pay a small premium that may include benefits beyond what is covered under the original Medicare program.

Network Adequacy Standards

VA and TRICARE use different standards for establishing provider networks. VA uses two key access standards:

> (i) geographic accessibility to a provider based on drive times, and (ii) appointment availability. Where access is inadequate (drive time or appointment availability) as determined by VA, the Contractor will be required to recruit providers and practitioners currently practicing in that area to participate in the [Community Care Network]. (VA, 2016)

VA's drive-time metric requires providers to be 30–60 minutes (primary care) or 45–180 minutes (general) drive time from a veteran's residence, depending on whether the veteran lives in a rural location. VA also sets maximum wait times for appointments of one day for emergent, two days for urgent, and 30 days for routine care.

DoD uses a network adequacy standard based on the concentration of providers inside and outside its TRICARE Prime service areas, which are the areas immediately near large military installations or with sizable beneficiary populations. DoD gives the TPA the flexibility to adjust the network according to the changing demands of enrollees, particularly if a base closes or a unit deploys: "All network providers . . . shall be sufficient in number, mix, and geographic distribution to provide the full scope of benefits for which all Prime enrollees are eligible under this contract" (DHA, 2016).

The private sector has moved toward very flexible network standards that are generally designed to fit the needs of the particular employer. Interviews with representatives from large benefits consulting firms and current and former DoD/VA TPAs indicated that TPAs generally estimate the potential demand for types of services and providers using demographic characteristics of the enrolled population, as well as the locations of providers and their specialty types. Other governmental programs, such as Medicare (through Medicare Advantage), have more formal network requirements for participating commercial plans (CMS, 2018a). Medicare Advantage requires that plans include a prespecified per capita (per Medicare beneficiary) number of providers in each county. CMS uses five density categories—large metropolitan, metro, micropolitan, rural, and counties with extreme access conditions—and the minimum number of providers varies by population density and specialty. CMS imposes adequacy requirements on 27 physician specialty types and 23 facility specialty types. It also requires that Medicare Advantage plans include a sufficient number of in-network providers to ensure that at least 90 percent of Medicare Advantage enrollees can access each provider type within predetermined distance and travel time standards. CMS establishes different travel-time and distance requirements based on county population density. The time and distance standards are calculated separately for each county and specialty combination. For example, primary care providers must be within a ten-minute drive or five-mile distance in large metro counties and within a 70-minute drive or 60-mile distance in a county with extreme access limits (very low-population-density counties) (CMS, 2018b).

Provider Payment Rates

It is difficult to know to what extent provider payment rates differ in practice between DoD and VA, because even though rates for both are based on Medicare, the actual rates may vary by geographic area and provider type (and this information was not shared with RAND). The VA MISSION Act sets Medicare payment rates as the standard rate.[4] This could affect the TPAs' leverage to gain discounts in return for increased volume in geographic areas with large numbers of veterans. DoD generally pays the Civilian Health and Medical Program of the Uniformed Services maximum allowable charge, which is defined as the 80th percentile of the charges for a given service nationwide, adjusted using Medicare's geographic adjustment factors. In some cases, the payment for particular services is set at Medicare rates (MHS, undated[c]).

Many (more than half of the 39) individuals we interviewed thought a potential benefit of a joint contract would be savings generated from lower provider payment rates in return for higher volume.

---

[4]   Section 101 of the VA MISSION Act "would establish payment rates for community care as, to the extent practicable, the Medicare rate" (Public Law 115-182).

However, if the payment rates are codified in legislation, and it is impossible for the TPAs to predict demand on the VA side, then it is unlikely that significant savings will be achieved through lower provider payment rates.

Sharing Medical Documentation Through a Joint Electronic Health Records Platform

DoD and VA face two problems in securely sharing medical information: sharing medical information between the departments and sharing medical information with community providers contracted in the purchased care network. Currently, DoD and VA operate separate electronic health records systems for their direct care facilities and providers. DoD is in the process of moving to Cerner's electronic health records (EHR) platform (what it calls MHS GENESIS) (MHS, undated[f]). VA currently uses a government-developed solution called VistA (VA, 2017c), which it has developed over the past three decades, but is also transitioning to the commercial Cerner EHR platform. More than half of our interviewees raised having a shared EHR as an operational issue for a joint contract and cited the difficulties that DoD and VA have faced in achieving this as a sign of the disparate cultures and working relationships that would need to be resolved to pursue a joint purchased care contract.

While a shared EHR would facilitate continuity of care for service members who transition to veteran status and for any beneficiary of either department who may receive care at an MTF or a VAMC, a joint EHR is not directly related to a joint contract with a TPA. TPAs do not mandate that providers use a particular EHR system. In theory, TPAs could mandate EHR use among their providers; however, they would likely not do so to encourage as many providers as possible to join and remain in their network.[5] DHA and VHA are not alone in their

---

[5] Alternatively, DoD or VA could pay for the software and hardware necessary to have purchased care providers use the DoD or VA EHR systems and provide this is as government-furnished equipment under the contracts for TRICARE and VA Community Care, respectively. However, the costs for these additional licenses and hardware are unknown, and this has not been incorporated into either department's TPA contracts by the contracting offices responsible for the respective programs.

struggle to share sensitive health information between different EHR systems. We note that this is an issue for the U.S. health care system as a whole and that a more efficient solution would be for the federal government to set standards for EHR interoperability to facilitate the sharing of medical records.

Each department's managed care support contracts (T2017 for DoD and PC3/Choice for VA) require medical documentation to be provided back to the departments for integration into beneficiary health records, but this does not uniformly occur via electronic means, nor does it give purchased care providers visibility into the EHRs maintained by each department's direct care system. DoD and VA senior leaders described an objective state in which their direct care and purchased care providers were able to share EHRs data across both the public/private divide and DoD/VA divide. However, there do not appear to be plans to pursue this objective state in the immediate future.

Interviewees reported that VA requires additional paperwork for participating providers, such as a requirement that providers submit relevant medical record information to VA providers. Several (between ten and 15 of the 39) interviewees noted that the paperwork requirements for providers who care for veterans in the community are far and above what is required from other payers. These interviewees noted that it is difficult to entice providers to participate in the VA network, other than for patriotism reasons, when providers must accept lower payment for more work. They also noted that providers often do not distinguish between active-duty service members and veterans in practice, considering them all part of the military. Furthermore, if office staff do not understand the difference in these requirements up front, it can cause delays in payment. (Until recently, VA community providers could not be paid until relevant medical record documentation was received.) Interviewees felt that standards for what information is shared with DoD or VA medical centers should be harmonized so that the same information is reported for both active-duty service members and veterans.

Incentive Structures

Both contracts have detailed performance incentives and reporting requirements for TPAs that would need to be harmonized to create economies of scale in administering the contracts. The TRICARE contracts have performance incentives for customer service (such as the percentage of phone calls to the help center that are answered within 30 seconds), fraud elimination, consumer satisfaction, claims processing turnaround times, and more. The TRICARE contracts also have incentives for TPAs to control spending by securing discounts from providers, decreasing the use of out-of-network care, and keeping total costs below national cost trends. VA's new RFP has fewer incentives than the TRICARE contracts, but they reflect some of the same performance metrics related to customer service, claims processing times, and limiting out-of-network care, so it is likely that the incentive and reporting requirements could be easily harmonized.

Representatives from current and former TPAs noted that the reporting requirements for both departments are well beyond the requirements in the private sector but may not be so uncommon among governmental programs. CMS, for example, requires that Medicare Advantage plans report annual information on (1) utilization, accessibility, and acceptability of services; (2) enrollee health status; (3) operational costs; and (4) other miscellaneous matters, as required. They are also required to submit encounter data (the managed care version of claims data) on an ongoing basis.

Potential to Incorporate Industry Practices

According to TRICARE, value-based purchasing is "any purchasing practices aimed at improving the value of health care services, where value is a function of both quality and cost" (AHRQ, 2002). In the private sector, value-based purchasing includes incentives for health plans, providers, and consumers: incentives for health plans or TPAs to improve the quality of care delivered, financial arrangements with providers to improve quality, and incentives for consumers to use higher-value services. Both DoD's current TRICARE contracts and VA's new

RFP direct TPAs to use industry best practices for care and disease management, utilization management, and population health management. We previously discussed the challenges associated with incentivizing the TPAs for quality reporting activities in the VA context, so we do not discuss them here. In this section, we examine the second and third approaches: value-based arrangements with providers and insurance design for consumers.

Value-Based Purchasing

Value-based purchasing is a term used to describe various initiatives that pay providers for improved quality or even patient outcomes. This largely involves payers and providers creating financial agreements to reward or sometimes penalize providers for care delivered to an enrolled population. At the time of this writing, DoD planned to allow its TPAs to begin experimenting with some of these pay-for-performance arrangements in 2018 (DoD, 2017b).

This is an area of ongoing innovation. Primary care medical homes, accountable care organizations, and value-based purchasing are examples of initiatives to pay providers in some way to increase quality. The programs can range from incentives for meeting quality benchmarks to arrangements in which providers may face penalties for not meeting quality standards. The CMS has experimented with a number of these programs, such as the Hospital Value-Based Purchasing program (CMS, 2018c), the Comprehensive Primary Care Plus model test (CMS, 2018d), and the Quality Payment Program (CMS, undated). All these programs are designed to financially reward providers for improved quality.

One of the more robust value-based purchasing experiments was Medicare's Pioneer Accountable Care Organization model test, in which CMS realigned payment incentives for certain experienced provider groups so that they would be based on better managed patient care rather than procedure volume. Starting with 32 accountable care organizations (ACOs) in 2012, the initial results showed the spending increased slightly less for Medicare beneficiaries enrolled in an ACO than for similar beneficiaries who received care from community providers (Nyweide et al., 2015). Early studies also showed modest savings for high-risk beneficiaries who tended to use more medical services (Colla et al., 2016).

There are two points of caution for any payer, including DoD or VA, that seeks to establish value-based payment arrangements. The first is that providers have to be willing to take on financial risk. This means that the provider group must be of sufficient size and have a reasonable level of technological sophistication to undertake population health management activities (Chukmaitov et al., 2017). The population for which the provider is responsible must be relatively stable and large enough; providers are unlikely to tolerate being financially penalized for populations of patients who may see multiple providers or live in an area for a short period. The instability of patient populations was flagged as an challenge to the Pioneer ACO program (Hsu et al., 2016). As such, provider groups that are willing to enter into risk arrangements will be available only in selected geographic markets for either VA or DoD, where the provider groups feel that they have the ability to take on the risk arrangements successfully (Chukmaitov et al., 2017). Although selected provider groups might willing to take on some financial risk, this will not be a widespread solution for reducing costs at this juncture for either DoD or VA.

Benefit Design

Much private-sector innovation in health insurance contracts is occurring around insurance benefit design and has focused on consumer— rather than provider—incentives to use higher-value care. Insurance benefit design addresses the services that are covered, the providers who are in the network, and the associated cost sharing for these services (deductibles, copayments, and coinsurance).

Health plans are also experimenting with adjusting patient cost sharing to steer utilization toward higher-value drugs, services, and even providers and steer patients away from services that are considered to be lower-value, also known as value-based insurance design (Robinson, Brown, and Whaley, 2017; Chernew, Rosen, and Fendrick, 2007). Health plans can exclude coverage for certain services or drugs altogether to reduce costs on these items or to drive utilization toward lower-cost, higher-value services. One example is a narrow network plan, which works by restricting the number of in-network providers (Gruber and McKnight, 2016; KFF, 2017). While narrow networks allow health plans to negotiate lower provider payments, they inherently limit the patient's choice of provider.

The National Defense Authorization Act for FY 2017 (Pub. L. 114-328) called for a value-based insurance design pilot program in TRICARE. It states that the DoD pilot will

> demonstrate and assess the feasibility of incorporating value-based health care methodology in the purchased care component of the TRICARE program by reducing co-payments or cost shares for targeted populations of covered beneficiaries in the receipt of high-value medications and services and the use of high-value providers under such purchased care component, including by exempting certain services from deductible requirements.

While DoD has been granted authority to experiment with value-based insurance design, VA is restricted by law from conducting these types of experiments with patient cost sharing.

Summary

TPAs conduct a variety of functions for payers (primarily employers) that can be sorted into two broad categories: (1) administrative functions related to enrollment, claims adjudication, customer service, and maintaining a network of providers and (2) additional services, such as providing recommendations on benefit design, utilization management services, population health monitoring, and care or disease management services.

The role of TRICARE TPAs is similar to that of TPAs in the private sector. The role of VA TPAs is to maintain a provider network, pay providers, provide customer service, and coordinate the sharing of medical record documentation between network providers and VA direct care facilities. There are other differences in the roles of these TPAs—for example, the scope of medical services that they manage, whether they coordinate with providers to sort the distribution of direct and purchased care, whether they manage the full spectrum of utilization for beneficiaries (similar to an employer health plan), and the extent to which they process claims. These differences could indicate barriers to integrating DoD and VA's purchased care contracting functions.

Both DoD and VA ask TPAs to report on some of the same quality metrics used by commercial and Medicare Advantage plans and have directed their TPAs to use industry best practices to manage utilization. However, the ability of VA TPAs to perform these functions remains limited because they do not see the majority of most veterans' care. This is an ongoing challenge for VA that would not be resolved by a joint contract.

Other challenges that would need to be addressed include claims processing procedures, provider payment rates, medical record sharing, and incentive structures for the departments' respective TPAs.

CHAPTER SIX

Potential Impact on Patients and Providers

Assuming that DoD and VA decide that an integrated purchased care approach is feasible and are able to resolve their operational differences, implementing integrated purchased care could have an effect on patients' and providers' experiences of care. We begin this chapter with opinions from interviewees regarding the potential impact of integration on patients and providers in terms of access to care, quality of care, and beneficiary experience. Then, we explore the potential impact on network size and characteristics if the existing provider networks were combined into an integrated network.

Potential Impact on Patients

Without conducting a specific pilot or demonstration, it is difficult to assess with certainty the effect that an integrated purchased care approach would have on patient experiences. Thus, we relied heavily on our interviewees' perspectives on how such an approach might affect purchased care access, quality, and costs, as well as satisfaction with purchased care among DoD beneficiaries and VHA-enrolled patients. These interview discussions were guided by our own expertise of how each health care system operates, and we used this expertise to inform the dialogue and ensure that interviewees were informed of the relevant nuances and distinctions to facilitate their responses. As necessary, we provided an overview of how DoD and VHA currently purchase care, whom they serve, and how they are financed to help ensure that interviewee comments and opinions are considered in the appropriate context. In total, we spoke with 39 individuals and asked them about their perceptions about how an integrated purchased care approach would affect patient experiences.

Access to Care

There was a common perception among those we spoke to that a joint contract would include a provider network that could be used by either DoD or VA beneficiaries. In general, interviewees thought that if a robust network were developed, access to care should improve for the entire population, particularly if patients were geographically dispersed. A few interviewees added that VA's experience with telehealth could further expand access. However, some (between six and nine of the 39) stated that there would still be access problems in some rural areas, where there are simply not enough providers to meet the demand for services. In addition, some (between six and nine of the 39) interviewees thought it was possible that TRICARE beneficiaries and VA enrollees would compete for some services, and, therefore, access would decline. This sentiment was expressed in both directions, with perceptions that either veterans or DoD beneficiaries would be squeezed out. One recent study that examined the potential impact of the ACA on TRICARE did find that demand from newly insured patients would motivate providers to alter their participation in TRICARE, thus providing some evidence of that expanded access and coverage could lead to changes in provider willingness to see patients (Mulcahy et al., 2017).

Quality of Care

Interviewees had mixed views of the impact of an integrated purchased care approach on quality. A few (between two and five of the 39) thought that, with more powerful contracting leverage, the new system could attract more high-quality providers—that is, if the new contract required building a new network to serve both departments simultaneously. Others expressed skepticism that quality would change, given that community providers nationally are criticized for using evidence-based practice at low rates and lacking cultural competence in working with military populations. (Many cited "RAND reports" that compare quality of care between VA and the private sector.) New providers might need to learn not only about military culture but also about the other health resources available to beneficiaries through DoD and VA. A few (between two and five of the 39) interviewees discussed how improved continuity of care—both within the treatment window for an illness and over time and across transitions from military service to veteran status—could be improved in an integrated system.

Other Patient-Level Factors

Other patient experiences mentioned by interviewees that could be affected by integration were scattered and tended to be anecdotal impressions. For instance, interviewees mentioned that a veteran might not wish to seek care from a TRICARE provider due to confidentiality concerns; a patient might become confused about access, benefits, and the need for authorization; or patients accustomed to VA care would experience shorter visits with less case management.

Other Relevant Data on Patient Perspectives

In addition to gathering insights from stakeholders on patients' preferences for where they receive care, we reviewed available reports from surveys. Patient preferences regarding where they receive care (either from a VA provider or the community) could inform the potential changes in demand within and across markets if the number of providers was suddenly expanded under a joint purchased care contract. For example, a membership survey conducted by the Veterans of Foreign Wars (VFW), a membership organization of veterans who were honorably discharged after serving in a war on foreign soil, provides some limited insights on veteran members' preferences in health care that may be relevant to consider in changing the approach to purchasing care (VFW, 2018). These data, from an online survey conducted in early 2018, are described as representative of the VFW's 1.2 million members. The sample was composed mostly of Vietnam-era veterans (60 percent) followed by Desert Storm–era veterans (26 percent) and post-9/11 veterans (25 percent).[1] Most of the veterans surveyed

---

[1]   Note that these are not mutually exclusive categories. For example, some Desert Storm–era veteran respondents may also be post-9/11 veterans if they served in both periods. Data

described satisfaction with VA care, with 80 percent saying they would recommend care to fellow veterans. Most relevant to the topic of purchased care, 59 percent of veterans who responded to the survey and had been offered community care chose to stay within VA, and 52 percent of veterans who were VA-eligible and also had private health insurance said they preferred to receive their care from VA. In addition, VFW members reported that VA providers understand their service-connected conditions better than private health care providers and spend more time with them than do private providers. In an earlier VFW survey from 2017, responding veterans identified quality of care as the most important factor when choosing a provider (79 percent), with availability of an appointment second (44 percent), and other factors related to convenience and cost less frequently endorsed (VFW, 2017).

With respect to TRICARE beneficiaries, there are some data from the annual TRICARE beneficiary survey to indicate that purchased care users rate their care more highly than TRICARE Prime users (who depend largely on direct care) based on the following metrics: get needed care (82 percent of non–TRICARE Prime purchased care users versus 71 percent TRICARE Prime users reported that they got needed care), get care quickly (86 percent versus 75 percent), doctor's communication (93 percent versus 90 percent), and customer service (80 percent versus 77 percent) (TRICARE, 2018b).

Potential Expansion of Provider Choice

One assertion that more than half of interviewees made was that an integrated purchased care approach would lead to a larger provider network by combining the existing networks for both departments. This assumes that a TPA would be able to leverage existing networks for the

---

on the representativeness of VFW members with respect to the overall characteristics of veterans of these foreign wars using VHA care was not available.

two departments and to the extent there is not overlap already, convince providers to join the new combined network.[2]

To examine the implications of integrating the existing two networks and to explore the extent of the current overlap between the two departments, we merged the individual-level provider data we received from each. As described in Chapter Three, these data included provider location (office address) and specialty. We combined the two provider lists and examined what a potential combined provider network would look like if the existing networks were simply added together. In this exercise, we assumed that the current TRICARE and VA networks meet current requirements and are adequate to meet the needs of their respective covered populations. This assumption is more likely to be reasonable for TRICARE, a well-established and stable program, than for VA, whose community care purchases have been increasing under the community care program. Utilization of purchased care is anticipated to continue to expand once new regulations resulting from the VA MISSION Act are implemented. We did not assess whether the existing networks, or the merging of them, would be sufficient to meet the needs of a combined TRICARE/VA population.

In reviewing the following analysis, it is important to note that providers typically contract to be in plan networks through groups, sometimes large, multispecialty groups. The provider data we received listed individual providers but did not identify the group through which each provider contracts. Therefore, we can provide only a rough idea of the potential gains in provider contracting costs in a combined network.

To get an idea of the increase in provider availability for TRICARE and VA beneficiaries, we measured the percentage increase in the number of network providers for each group in each county in the United States. We used counties to approximate health care market areas. We found that simply combining the two existing provider networks would increase the number of network providers for TRICARE

---

[2]   At least in the short term, we assume that a TPA would offer contracts to the preexisting network first and then fill in where necessary with additional providers, since this would preserve continuity of care for beneficiaries.

and VA in most counties, at least for some specialty groups. The benefit of this network expansion is unclear. With the data available for this study, we could not assess whether patients would experience more timely appointments, be able to choose providers they prefer, or benefit from higher quality care. To the extent that these benefits occur, it is likely that the demand for purchased care will increase, especially among veterans. More providers contracting to be in the VA network may mean that more patients seek VA services instead of services paid through other coverage (e.g., employer plan, Medicaid, Medicare). The same could be true for TRICARE beneficiaries, but they already primarily rely on TRICARE.

Across all specialties, the increase in the number of providers in a combined network varies by the type of county for both TRICARE and VA (Figure 6.1). By merging the two current lists of providers, the network of available providers to serve TRICARE beneficiaries would expand more in rural areas than in urban areas; the network would increase by about 25 percent in large metro areas and by just over 50 percent in more rural areas. The pattern for VA patients is reversed. Provider availability would increase by 35–40 percent in more rural areas and more than double in large metro areas. These results are consistent with the assumption that the current networks reflect the needs of the respective beneficiary populations for purchased care, at least under current policy. For example, the TRICARE network is designed to have a concentration of providers near MTFs, which are primarily in more urban areas, while the VHA network has more rural providers to meet the needs of veterans living in rural areas. Merging the two existing networks potentially expands the number providers to serve beneficiaries of either system but it still does not indicate whether the network would be adequate or sufficient to meet the needs of both populations. This exercise does not assess whether a TPA operating a joint contract would decide to build a network by merging the existing provider networks for both departments.[3]

---

[3] A TPA could instead build a network by starting with its existing provider network for other payers. However, given that the TRICARE and VA network terms and beneficiary locations are different from those of a typical commercial payer, we would not expect sig-

Figure 6.1
Percentage Increase in TRICARE Versus VA Providers, by County Type
(median across counties of each type)

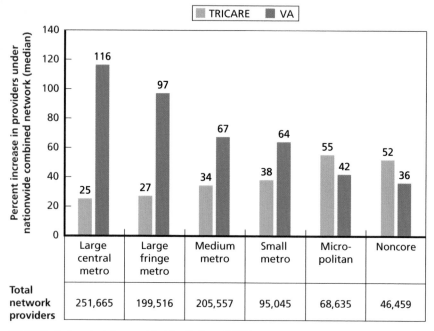

SOURCE: Network data provided by DoD and VHA.

Measuring the increase in the number of providers within a specialty group in a county was challenging because many counties have few or no providers in either the TRICARE or VA network. Figure 6.2 shows the percent increase in the TRICARE and VA networks for each specialty group for all counties combined. The figure excludes pediatrics specialties because VA almost never treats children. The VA network would expand much more than the TRICARE network for all specialties except the adult specialties group, which includes medical subspecialists and surgical specialists. VA has a robust network of adult specialists because so many of its patients are older or have a

nificant overlap with existing commercial networks, although we were unable to assess this directly.

Figure 6.2
Nationwide Percentage Increase in TRICARE Versus VA Providers, by Specialty Group

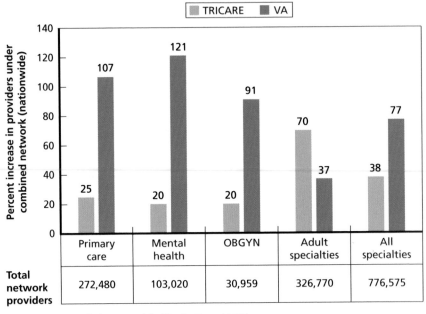

SOURCE: Network data provided by DoD and VHA.

disability. The TRICARE population, which is younger and healthier, requires less of this type of care.

Further evaluation of the potential gains from combining the TRICARE and VA networks would require an analysis of the purchased care utilization by TRICARE and VA patients as a function of their access to direct care services. This analysis would need to be done at the local level to make useful connections between beneficiary demand, in-house capability, and purchased care. The analysis would also have to consider that VA care purchases may not have reached a steady state under current policy. As noted previously, many enrolled veterans rely on VA for only some of their care, but the history of TRICARE suggests that putting in place a robust network to supplement care in VA facilities would shift their reliance to VA over time. As we discuss in the next chapter, as VA extends opportunities to get more care in the community, it is likely that more enrolled veterans would begin using their VA health care benefit and those already using VA health care would rely on it more. Therefore, the more extensive analysis outlined here would have to be repeated as demand and utilization change.

Potential Impact on Participating Providers

Interviewees discussed several possible impacts on providers in an integrated system of purchased care. Under a joint contract, providers would have to decide whether to participate. Some interviewees expressed concern that because the paperwork requirements for VA providers are so different than the requirements for VA, TRICARE providers may not want to join a unified network. Some (between six and ten of the 39) mentioned shifts in expectations from the current systems—for instance, that TRICARE providers might be hesitant to share patient records in the way that VA has required to date, or that providers have been frustrated with slow payments from VA and might expect the same within an integrated network, which could lead providers to be unwilling to participate. Data from the Veterans Choice Program Provider Satisfaction Survey showed that community providers who had delivered care to veterans through Veterans Choice were less than fully satisfied with their experience, which could affect their decision to participate in a new, joint contract. In the survey, community providers who delivered care through Veterans Choice were asked to rate their satisfaction with Health Net or TriWest staff members, processes, and how problems and complaints were handled (VA, 2017d). Approximately 632 respondents participated in the 2017 survey; more than 54 percent used services from Health Net and 46 percent used services from TriWest. Overall, 58 percent had experienced a problem in the previous three months, and only half of respondents reported that they were satisfied with TPA services, including receiving error-free payments in a timely manner (45 percent were satisfied), authorizations for care (50 percent), and billing (48 percent). However, more than two-thirds (68 percent) stated that they had necessary patient information and documentation to provide care to veteran patients in time for their appointment, and 85 percent reported that they would use their contractor's services again and continue to provide services to veterans.

Interviewees mentioned that a potential benefit of a joint contract for participating providers would be having one set of administrative processes and for providers to become part of the network for both departments. For example, a few (fewer than five of the 39) interviewees stated that providers do not necessarily distinguish the TRICARE and VA purchased care programs and find it confusing that they face more requirements and paperwork for veteran visits as opposed to military personnel visits.

Some (between six and ten of the 39) respondents suggested that a joint contract could be very confusing for a provider if they had to sort out the various benefits and eligibility requirements, but others noted that if it were a single system with benefits managed by the TPA, this process could become easier for providers. Some (six of 39) interviewees talked about an integrated network being favorable in terms of maintaining credentials in subspecialties, but these comments seemed to focus more on direct care, such as trauma surgery.

Summary

A decision to pursue an integrated purchased care approach could have implications for both providers and patients. We spoke with 39 stakeholders to get their impressions of what such an approach might look like and to gain a better understanding of the potential effects on participating providers and patient experiences.

There was a common perception among our interviewees that a joint contract would include a provider network that could be used by either DoD or VA beneficiaries and that a robust network should improve access to care for the entire population. However, several remained concerned about access for rural populations and thought it was possible that TRICARE beneficiaries and VA enrollees would compete for some services, thus decreasing access to care. There were also mixed views on the impact on quality.

Patients' preferences regarding where they receive care could inform the potential changes in demand within and across markets. Of a sample of veterans surveyed in early 2018, around half of those who were VA-eligible, also had private health insurance, and had been offered community care said they preferred to receive their care from VA. Surveyed veterans also noted that VA providers understood their service-connected conditions better than private health care providers and also spent more time with them. Among TRICARE beneficiaries, there is some evidence that purchased care users rate their care more highly than TRICARE Prime users (who depend largely on direct care) in terms of timeliness and quality.

With the data available for this study, we could not assess whether patients would experience more timely appointments, be able to choose providers they prefer, or benefit from higher-quality care. However, we were able to estimate the potential increase in the number of providers under an integrated purchased care approach, finding that it would vary by the type of county for both TRICARE and VA. Further evaluation of the potential gains from combining the TRICARE and VA networks would require an analysis of purchased care utilization by TRICARE and VA patients as a function of their access to direct care services.

Stakeholder perspectives on the impact on providers were mixed, with interviewees expressing concern about an increased paperwork burden for TRICARE providers, a potential reluctance among TRICARE providers to share patient records, payment delays when providing care through VA, and possible procedural and administrative challenges that could vary depending on how the networks are integrated.

CHAPTER SEVEN

Potential Impact on Costs

As DoD and VA weigh whether an integrated purchased care approach will yield any potential cost savings for the government, we highlight a few categories of costs that should be examined as part of this decisionmaking process.

TPA Administrative Costs of Managing the Contracts

The two departments should consider the extent to which policies can be harmonized to lower administrative costs for TPAs. As described in Chapter Five, there are considerable differences in operational processes for TPAs between the two departments, such as differences in provider contracting, claims processing, reporting, and customer service functions. If the departments maintain separate standards for any of these major functions, then there are fewer efficiencies to be gained from a joint purchased care contract. There could be savings if the departments can negotiate a lower fee and overhead paid to the TPA for conducting these activities in a joint contract.

Provider Credentialing and Contracting

A combined provider network could be expected to lower the duplicative contracting costs for the two departments to the extent that some of the same providers currently contract separately with both networks. However, the efficiency gain from jointly contracting for network providers depends on how similar the network requirements are by location and specialty for TRICARE and VA, as well as the requirements to enroll as a provider. Complementary, rather than overlapping, networks would still require the same number of providers to contract with the departments. Any lingering differences, such as one department requiring more documentation to enroll as a provider, would reduce the potential efficiency gains in streamlining the contracting process.

Provider Payments

The main costs associated with both contracts are payments to providers per service. Both DoD and VA pay for services on a fixed-price or cost-type basis, but the actual payments may differ between the departments. While both use Medicare as a benchmark, VA, for example, may pay more than this rate for an individual provider in a rural area.

Many respondents noted that a joint network could achieve savings through the ability to lower payments to providers. Theoretically, the combined volume of visits could be leveraged to negotiate discounts with providers. However, there are factors that could prevent a joint contract actually producing savings from lower payments to providers. The first is that both DoD and VA pay near Medicare rates, and it is not clear that providers would be willing to take lower rates, particularly given other studies demonstrating the potential impact of the ACA on TRICARE participation (Mulcahy et al., 2018). Second, VA is not able to anticipate its demand for community services in a way that would allow the TPAs to use these data in negotiations with providers. If the TPAs cannot accurately judge the volume of predicted services, they cannot use this as leverage in negotiations with providers. Finally, negotiating lower rates in return for increased volume requires that the departments be able to steer patients to these preferred providers through either lower cost sharing or an HMO-style plan that limits the choice of providers. TRICARE is limited in its ability to do this under the Select plan (which is similar to a PPO, with fairly unrestricted choice), and both agencies are legally limited in their use of copayments as a tool to steer patients to certain providers.

Potential Impact on Costs to Government

Interviewees indicated that an integrated purchased care approach might bring about some efficiencies and economies of scale on the government side, which would lead to lower management costs for both departments, particularly VA. VA currently has a significantly larger staff managing its community care contracts in comparison to DoD, according to our review of organizational charts for the two departments. However, we note that some of this difference could be explained by the departments' use of contracted management services. VHA currently requires 7,287 full-time equivalent (FTE) employees to manage the community care programs. The bulk of the FTEs are devoted to claims adjudication and reimbursement (2,279 FTEs) and revenue operations (3,744) (VA, 2018a). In contrast, DoD has approximately 230 FTEs working as part of the TRICARE health plan and an additional 350–400 FTEs managing other aspects of the process, for a total of approximately 580–630 FTEs total.[1]

Interviewees thought that savings might come primarily from reduced DHA and VHA staff time to manage duplicative processes across both departments. For example, if VA were to allow its TPAs to take on the role of claims adjudication, there are potentially larger savings in reduced staff time to manage this process. However, a few also pointed out that the complexity of benefits management and authorizations might wash out some of the efficiencies, or that there might be additional unanticipated costs. One person suggested that any cost savings should be rolled over into training and quality assurance practices, and another assumed that there would be an increase in cost to government. Finally, managing a joint contract may require additional staff at the clinic or hospital level to serve as liaisons with a larger contractor.

Changes in Utilization

An integrated purchased care approach may affect costs in other ways, too. Evidence suggests that new programs of care, particularly those that affect access, can affect veterans' reliance on and utilization of VA

---

[1] Personal communication with a TRICARE health plan representative, June 2018.

health care (Hebert et al., 2018; Eibner et al., 2015). If access under the joint contract improves, more beneficiaries—particularly veterans without TRICARE eligibility—may be likely to use the purchased care system and rely more heavily overall on VA for their care. That, in turn, may change the amount of money required to deliver health care to meet increased demand. Increasing utilization of VA purchased care could also have downstream effects on VHA's other missions of education and research; as more veterans seek care from the community rather than VA facilities, there could be fewer opportunities and resources for provider training within VA facilities and research programs focused on veterans' health care needs.

Out-of-pocket costs might also affect demand for services, most notably by moderating utilization if copayments rise. Because patient cost-sharing amounts for TRICARE and VHA are defined by legislation, interviewees generally thought that there would be little impact on patient out-of-pocket costs, under the assumption that benefits and eligibility would remain static with an integrated purchased care approach. However, a few (fewer than five of the 39) interviewees pointed out that the TPA for a joint contract may have difficulty charging veterans the correct copayments, which vary by priority enrollment group. Under VA's current statutory priority group scheme, veterans in the top priority group pay no copayments, and those in priority groups 2–8 pay varying levels of copayments based on whether the treatment is being provided for a service-connected condition, their priority group level, their means, and other factors. Thus, calculating the specific cost-sharing amount might seem complicated for the TPA if it has only limited information about the veteran's medical history. This system differs from the DoD TRICARE copayment structure, which more closely resembles that of a private-sector insurance plan. For providers who treat patients under a joint contract, there was concern among our interviewees about TRICARE providers inadvertently charging VA patients copayments that are not required or vice versa. In contrast, representatives from current and former TPAs, as well as benefits managers, felt that TPAs can easily administer different benefit designs for different groups as they currently do for large employers.

Summary

Several factors could influence whether an integrated approach to purchased care yields savings for the government. As DoD and VA assess the options moving forward, they should consider differences in TPAs' operational processes. For example, a combined provider network could be expected to lower the duplicative provider contracting costs, but the extent of these savings depends on how similar the network requirements are by location and specialty for TRICARE and VA and the requirements to enroll as a provider. Furthermore, the main costs associated with both contracts are payments to providers per service; both DoD and VA pay for services on a fixed-price or cost-type basis, but the actual payments may differ.

If access under a joint contract improves, more beneficiaries—particularly veterans without TRICARE eligibility—may be likely to use the purchased care system and rely more heavily on VA for their care. That, in turn, may change the amount of money required to deliver health care to meet increased demand. Changes to out-of-pocket costs might also affect demand for services. Differences between the VHA and TRICARE copayment structures also pose a challenge, and there were mixed opinions among interviewees about whether TPAs were equipped to handle cost sharing accurately.

CHAPTER EIGHT

Summary Observations and Recommendations

This chapter summarizes additional insights gleaned from our stakeholder interviews with respect to the overall challenges and considerations for the two departments as they evaluate their next steps in this process. We also provide a summary of the preliminary feasibility assessment and present recommendations for moving forward.

Stakeholder Suggestions

Individuals interviewed offered many comments with respect to how an integrated purchased care approach could be designed, the essential features it should have, and other factors that should be considered in moving forward.

Feasibility Depends on the Contract and Network Design

Multiple interviewees expressed ideas about the requirements for a high-functioning integrated purchased care approach. The consensus among those we spoke with was that a high-functioning system could be built but that "the devil is in the details." Interviewees mentioned several important considerations in setting up integrated purchased care, as summarized in Table 8.1. The left column lists the suggestions received from interviewees, and the right column provides relevant information from the RAND assessment to inform judgment of whether the suggestion is realistic or appropriate.

Table 8.1
Summary of Stakeholder Suggestions for Designing an Integrated Purchased Care Approach

Interviewee Suggestion	RAND Comment
Develop a robust, well-located provider network with the right mix of specialties, possibly several regional networks.	To create such a network, additional analyses will be necessary to more accurately predict and map demand to the available providers to determine where additional provider recruitment would be needed to ensure the "right" mix of capabilities and capacity.
Consider blended funding and ways to simplify reimbursements.	Without changes to legislation restricting the use of DoD and VHA funding or new legislation that specifically grants permission for a joint funding account, it is not possible to blend funding for a joint purchased care contract.
Prioritize quality (including a strong requirement for quality oversight, required training in military culture and specific military-related health problems, and, perhaps, demonstrated competencies prior to joining the network).	At present, each department interacts with and has different expectations for the role of its TPAs. VA TPAs are responsible for only a small portion of a veteran's overall care, and, as such, these expectations may be overly burdensome for what might amount to a very small volume of care. At present, DoD does not have these requirements for its TRICARE providers, so this would also represent a new contractual requirement that could limit provider willingness to participate.
Measure timeliness and outcomes and develop an associated system of accountability for providers, possibly a value-based system.	At present, DoD and VA have different expectations about the TPA's role in ensuring timeliness and measuring outcomes. Putting in place mechanisms to monitor and assess access and outcomes of care would require significant effort. While DoD has tried to implement more value-based purchasing approaches within TRICARE, it has done so by shifting some risk to the TPA. Within VA, implementing this approach could be much more challenging due to the current role of TPAs and regulations for how VA purchases care in the community.
Standardize referral processes, authorizations, credentialing, and privileging of providers, claims processing and reimbursements; this would best be implemented by using a single EHR system.	Addressing the differences in how DoD and VA handle these issues will require legislative, regulatory, and contractual changes to align many of the current differences in how they interact with TPAs, the processes they use for storing and sharing information between providers, and the requirements they have for authorizing/credentialing providers.

Table 8.1—Continued

Interviewee Suggestion	RAND Comment
Develop a mechanism to manage the complex benefit structure that differs for beneficiaries—some of whom have dual eligibility or service-connected disability benefits—possibly by using a single contractor that can manage the differing benefits as is done for different employer plans.	While TPAs do have experience managing different product lines, it is not clear that just having the same TPA manage the purchased care functions for both DoD and VA would achieve integration or yield any increased efficiency for the government.
Add flexibility to meet the changing needs of patient populations as demographics and health care preferences change, as well as changes in legislation on benefits and eligibility.	Specific contract mechanisms may be needed to allow changes to the requirements and funding to be made in response to such shifts or changes.
Use best industry standards and have an experienced management structure.	Both DoD and VA have designated offices that oversee their purchased care functions. Ensuring the appropriate workforce within these offices can facilitate the adoption and implementation of industry standards.
Have a strong customer service element.	Interviewees stressed the importance of customer service and pointed to problems that both DoD and VA have experienced in implementing changes to their purchased care programs, particularly with respect to how well the TPA communicated changes and handled questions. Any transition to a new network or major shift in the processes used for consumers to gain access to purchased care will require education and a focus on customer service.

Other Important Considerations for Designing an Effective Integrated Purchased Care Approach

Interviewees raised several other considerations as well, including issues related to governance, department culture, leadership, and policy oversight. The way each of these issues is addressed could have important implications for how effective an integrated purchased care approach would be.

Governance

In terms of governance, ideas ranged from a joint coalition to an integrated office to rotating authority. There are many significant structural and governance questions regarding the precise parameters of an integrated, joint contract for purchased care that remained unanswered at the conclusion of our study. For example,

- Which entity should own and administer the contract?
- To whom will this administrating entity report? How will interagency governance be achieved? What structural changes will need to be made to department structures (i.e., positions and titles of Senate-confirmed appointees and their offices) to manage this new contract?
- What cost-sharing or reimbursement mechanisms will be put in place to fund the contract? How will they work in conjunction with current DoD/VA appropriations, or will the appropriations be changed to fit the contract?
- What degree of integration will be sought between each department's direct care operations and to link the direct and purchased care operations across the two departments? To what extent will direct care and purchased care providers be obligated or encouraged to use a common EHR platform, or to adhere to other common reporting requirements?
- How will service members, veterans, and their families access a new, integrated network? Will there be one point of entry (e.g., website, call center, directory) or two (or more than two), depending on the type of beneficiary? Will beneficiaries be able to use a web-based portal for appointments or record management?

Should DoD and VA move forward with an integrated approach, these questions will require considerable attention.

Differences in Department Cultures

As noted earlier in this report, each of these federal health care systems was designed with a different primary mission. Each maintains its own facilities, separate workforces, and separate administrative processes for similar lines of operation in the health care arena. While some sharing does occur, including the sharing of facilities in specific pilot programs, most interviewees maintained that these systems and their workforces have largely different cultures. Notwithstanding the notion that DoD already has multiple cultures (e.g., for each branch of the military), this cultural distinction was often cited as a challenge to working together effectively.

Multiple interviewees underscored that DoD and VA's differing missions and cultures could pose challenges to an integrated purchased care approach. Historically, these mission and cultural differences have been somewhat hard to reconcile, and, thus, some interviewees expressed skepticism that this effort would be different. Others were skeptical of how integration could occur, given that DoD and VA have not worked well together in the past, and some interviewees were not convinced that they could manage this well. One commented that DoD usually "bigfoots" VA, and, often, VA does not know what it wants, leading to concern that it lacks the ability to administer an integrated contract.

In contrast to these views, a few interviewees pointed out the similarities in mission: Both departments seek to improve the health of people who at some point were in uniform, and both systems go outside the direct care system when necessary to ensure access or quality of services. One interviewee pointed out that taking care of veterans should be a key part of the DoD mission in terms of the perceptions of future recruits; however, there is little evidence to indicate whether this is a valid concern or how an integrated purchased care approach would affect individual decisions regarding military accession.

Leadership

Several (between ten and 15 of the 39) interviewees pointed out that the development of an integrated purchased care approach would require "a big lift" and, therefore, stable, engaged, and consistent leadership from VA, DoD, and Congress. One suggested that operational, strategic, and political leadership at the secretary (or deputy secretary) level would be necessary. Some (between six and nine of the 39) pointed out political challenges, such as that this initiative might be seen as part of controversial privatization of VA or as a sign that VA might reduce its footprint or close doors. Another pointed out the challenge of general inertia in government, slowing change. A few interviewees expressed concern about leadership on the VA side due to several recent departures of key leaders. Most interviewees pointed out that the leadership would need to be strong and committed to prevent backsliding.

Policy Oversight for Legislative and Regulatory issues

At present, there are four oversight committees in Congress that have a critical role in shaping policy and programs for how the departments furnish health care: the House and Senate Armed Services Committees and the House and Senate Veterans Affairs Committees. All have a vested interest in any considerations related to changes with respect to purchasing care for service members, military dependents, or veterans. Thus, they will each need to be consulted on alternative approaches. They will also serve a critical role in implementing any necessary changes to existing legal and regulatory authorities governing how the systems furnish (deliver and purchase) health care, including rules and restrictions on how federal funds are used across agencies. Coordination with the relevant appropriations committees in both the House and Senate would also be required.

Implications of the Evolving Policy Landscape

The past several years have been a time of significant change in how both DoD and VA furnish health care. For example, each department has been congressionally directed to make significant changes to how it manages and furnish health care. At the same time, there have been significant changes in the U.S. health care system that also affect DoD and VA. Thus, the decision to proceed must consider how this rapidly evolving landscape could directly affect the feasibility and effectiveness of an integrated purchased care approach. In this section, we discuss some of the ongoing policy changes and concerns that interviewees mentioned as being relevant.

Ongoing Policy Changes at DHA and VHA

In recent years, there have been major changes to TRICARE, as well as changes to how DoD manages its health care functions (i.e., creation and implementation of DHA). As oversight of MTF care management has shifted to DHA, DoD has also implemented new contracting timelines and requirements. Congress has required DoD to transform TRICARE's financial structure from a traditional "cost-plus" fee-for-service government contract to a "value-based" structure that reduces government costs and incentivizes contractors to generate better health outcomes for beneficiaries. The National Defense Authorization Act for FY 2017 directed DoD to move in this direction, and DoD's most recent TRICARE procurement contract (T2017) did so.

Similarly, there have been significant changes to how VA utilizes and manages purchased care. With the passage of the Veterans Choice Act in 2014, VA's use of care in the community became a focal point of national attention and debate, and VA subsequently experienced an increase in demand for care. While VA worked to create new management approaches for its community care programs, it continued to face external pressures to expand how veterans might get care in the community. Even prior to the passage of the VA MISSION Act, VA was working to improve its programs and change how it contracted for care in the community through its new Community Care Network contracts.

Adapting to these policy changes has taken time and resources within both departments, and, as such, any additional changes could disrupt ongoing efforts to implement prior policy changes.

Policy Changes to the External Health Care Market That Directly Affect Reliance on VA and TRICARE

As noted earlier, changes in the U.S. health care system overall also affect VA and DoD. This is particularly the case for VA. Changes in the health care policy landscape affect veterans' access to other sources of health insurance and thus affect their demand for VA services. Veterans may pick and choose where to receive care depending on their out-of-pocket payments, perceived quality of care, and ability to easily get an appointment if they have multiple sources of coverage (e.g., Medicare, employer-sponsored insurance). For example, if they are able to have prescriptions filled at VA for free or with minimal copays, they are more likely to do so rather than filling prescriptions at a community pharmacy and paying copayments. The ACA, which increased the availability of insurance among individuals without access to employer-sponsored coverage, is an example of the types of health reforms that would affect demand for purchased care accessed through VA and TRICARE (Dworsky et al., 2017; Mulcahy et al., 2017). While the ACA expanded coverage through Medicaid to childless adults, newer policies, such as work requirements to maintain coverage, may reduce eligibility for some veterans and increase their reliance on VA.

For TRICARE beneficiaries, the impact may be more nuanced. For active-duty service members and their dependents, these changes are likely to have little impact, and their demand for care is less likely to be influenced by non-DoD policy factors. For members of the reserve component, the ACA's individual mandate may have increased their reliance on TRICARE; however, the Tax Cuts and Jobs Act of 2017 (Pub. L. 115-97) eliminated mandate penalties starting in 2019. So, the incentives that the individual mandate previously created that led personnel to turn to TRICARE coverage may vanish. On the other hand, those who newly enrolled in TRICARE as a result of the mandate may stay enrolled well after the penalty is removed just due to inertia in making health care coverage changes. Beneficiaries who maintain benefits through military retirement or medical discharge may have additional options and sources of coverage. This may include employer-sponsored health insurance or eligibility for VA health care (Hepner et al., 2017; DoD, 2014). Expanded coverage for non-DoD beneficiaries through the ACA might also affect the willingness of TRICARE providers to remain engaged with TRICARE, particularly if TRICARE rates remain lower than Medicare or Medicaid rates (Mulcahy et al., 2017). For example, one study of the ACA's impact on TRICARE found that the infusion of newly insured patients could make private providers less likely to engage with TRICARE due to differences in payment amounts (Mulcahy et al., 2017).

Other External Factors That May Affect Feasibility

There will always be a focus on safety and quality within federal health systems, particularly for DoD and VA. Quality and safety concerns will always grab headlines when it comes to military and veteran populations and are likely to result in congressional responses that might change benefits, reporting requirements, and system design. However, TPAs may have limited capabilities to manage these issues if they are responsible for only a portion of an individual's care, such as in the case of the VA Community Care program. It is more reasonable to delegate responsibility and set expectations around safety, quality, and outcomes if the TPA is responsible for the total health of the covered population, as it is for TRICARE TPAs for a subset of the DoD beneficiary population.

It is also important to recognize that timely access to high-quality care is a national problem, but it is not limited to VA. MTFs have also had problems, and so has the private sector (Tanielian et al., 2018; Basu et al., 2012). The private sector is not always the "beacon of hope" for solving these issues. For example, an increasing number of health care providers have stopped participating in insurance networks or accepting any third-party reimbursement (Philpott, 2017; DoD, 2007). This shifts the burden onto the consumer to deal with bureaucratic processes and can raise their share of the cost. All these factors make maintaining an adequate network of providers a challenge.

Uncertainty of Future Demand

It should be noted that any changes that affect the size of the covered populations would also affect how an integrated purchased care approach would operate in practice. Current population projections suggest that the veteran population will continue to shrink over the next ten to 20 years as large World War II, Korea, Vietnam, and Cold War–era cohorts are replaced by smaller cohorts of younger veterans (Eibner et al., 2015). In another example, changes to eligibility for TRICARE or VA health care would likely affect the nature and volume of demand and drive changes to how the departments balance their delivery of health care services across their direct and purchased care programs. As any of those topics are considered (including restricting or unrestricting access to VHA by some priority enrollment groups), analyses will be needed to determine the resulting impact on utilization of services. Similarly, as U.S. troops engage in future deployments, particularly those that involve combat operations, we would expect shifts in the types and volume of care that would be required to address not only the potential casualties associated with those missions but also the demand among other beneficiary groups. This uncertainty could also create challenges to how DoD and VA would manage and utilize an integrated purchased care contract.

Conclusions

According to our review of the existing legal and regulatory authorities for DoD and VHA, an integrated purchased care approach (including a joint contract and shared list of providers) would be legally permissible; however, some changes to existing authorities would be required, specifically with respect to how current appropriations language refers to the relevant programs for purchasing care. From our review of the TPA contracts and interviews with stakeholders about how the departments utilize their purchased care contract, we identified significant concerns with respect to the operational practicality of an integrated purchased care contract. Many (more than half of the 39) interviewees noted that the "devil is in the details" and that, without significant changes in the way in which each department engages with the TPA (particularly for VA), any operational efficiencies would be limited. Our interviews also revealed an uncertain impact on patient experiences. Some (between six and nine of the 39) interviewees believed that an integrated approach to purchasing care could expand the number of providers available to both departments. While this point is partially supported by our finding that simply combining or merging lists of providers would increase the total number of providers "in network," it is important to note that if an integrated purchased care program were pursued through a joint contractor, the TPA (particularly if it were a new vendor to DoD or VA) would likely build a fresh list of network providers based on the parameters outlined in the RFP. It is not clear whether this would be a simple combination of old lists. As such, our analyses of the combined lists were unable to determine whether these expansions would fill gaps or be enough to reach network sufficiency for either department. Some (between six and nine of the 39) inter- viewees also thought that combining purchased care programs could create artificial competition between the two populations (TRICARE beneficiaries and VHA patients referred out to community care) for access to the same providers. Without information about the capacity of each of the providers and the potential demand for their services within an integrated purchased care program, it is difficult to assess the specific impact that such an approach would have on patient access.

Our examination of the potential impact on costs also yielded uncertainty. While some stakeholders believed that the government might be able to achieve greater cost-efficiency by negotiating lower payments to providers based on some expectation of increased volume of services, both departments are already paying near Medicare rates to their contracted providers. There could be some cost savings associ- ated with a joint purchased care contract through sharing of contract- ing functions and processes, however, but without the legal/regulatory changes in how those contracts are established, it might just be a matter of shifting costs from one department to the rather than a means of achieving any real savings to the government. Some (between six and nine of the 39) interviewees posited that there could be an increase in costs to the government from having to create additional oversight mechanisms to ensure that the joint contract still followed appropri- ate legislative, regulatory, and other legal requirements that govern the use of respective DoD and VHA funding. So, although the TPA rep- resentatives we spoke to indicated that they could handle setting up structures and processes to handle the distinctions between DoD and VA, they emphasized that, due to the very different approaches used by the departments to purchase care, they would still largely be managed independently as two different product lines.

Recommendations

Given the many uncertainties outlined here, we highlight two recommendations that aim to reduce some of the unknowns and provide concrete evidence of the impact that an integrated purchased care approach would have on costs, patient experiences, and operations within both departments. Ideally, these recommendations should be considered in parallel but implemented sequentially. The additional analyses outlined in the first recommendation would inform the design and implementation of a pilot or demonstration which is the focus of the second recommendation. Only a pilot or demonstration will provide concrete evidence to document the impact of an integrated purchased care approach on the departments, the populations they serve, and the government more broadly.

Conduct Additional Analyses

To further examine the feasibility and practicality of integrating purchased care, DoD and VA could consider pursuing additional analyses that use individual-level data on the demand for purchased care across both departments to examine similarities and differences. The analyses could examine trends within regions or among specific populations. Overlaying the results with analyses of the provider networks would offer a more robust understanding of whether an integrated purchased care approach would help improve provider access for each department.

Further analyses for merging contracting functions could also explore specific staffing capabilities and needs across the two departments, identifying where positions and responsibilities align or where they require independent approaches.

Should the departments wish to move forward in integrating their purchased care functions, additional analyses will also be needed to explore the various options for oversight. There are many issues to resolve with respect to how a joint oversight function would work and likely advantages and disadvantages, as well as differing costs, associated with the various options.

Design, Implement, and Evaluate a Pilot or Demonstration Project
To clarify the potential impact of an integrated purchased care system, some interviewees suggested that the departments consider designing and implementing a series of pilots or demonstrations. In our interviews, senior leaders thought that standing up this type of integrated purchased care approach might take between five and ten years, and several suggested that implementation should start small, perhaps with some pilots or focused on a specific type of health care, to pave the way for full integration down the road.

Using their respective demonstration authorities, the departments could collaborate with Congress to outline the parameters for one or more demonstration (pilot) efforts for integrating different dimensions of purchased care across DoD and VA. While there are multiple variations and levels of integration that could be considered, tested, and evaluated in such a pilot, several (ten to 15 of the 39) individuals we spoke to suggested that it would be important to choose a specific geographic region or market, or perhaps to identify a specific type of health care service (e.g., adult specialty services) or type of health care provider (e.g., OB/GYN) to examine how integration might affect access, costs, and quality of care.

Figure 8.1 provides a notional, illustrative step ladder toward greater integration. This notional spectrum of integration was devised solely for discussion purposes with the sponsor to outline how different parts of an integrated purchased care approach could be considered in a building-block fashion in that each step would require additional levels of intervention with respect to regulatory/legal, operational, and governance changes. As a first step, for example, DoD and VA could consider simply sharing lists of providers by requiring their TPAs to exchange relevant information on providers or to facilitate expedited contracting for both departments. The second step would involve the two departments working to consolidate or compile their requirements

Figure 8.1
Illustrative Integration "Step" Ladder

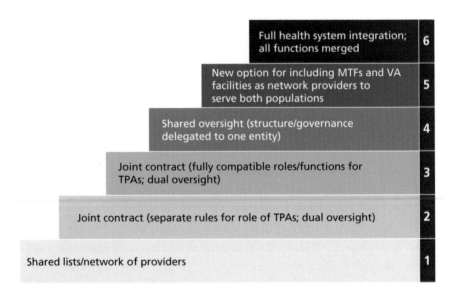

for purchased care networks into a single contract mechanism that outlines two different sets of rules, functions, and roles for two separate programs. Additional steps would involve increasing amounts of integration. At the highest level, it would include integrating all functions within both health systems.

Under one or more demonstration projects, DoD and VA could work with Congress to establish specific governance approaches and funding mechanisms to address the issues surrounding oversight, use of different funding streams, and contracting terms. Several (between ten and 15 of the 39) interviewees indicated that prior experiences with resource sharing (e.g., EHR integration, facility sharing in North Chicago) might yield important insights for how these demonstrations would be established, including how best to avoid prior barriers to integrating functions across the two departments.

Summary

Our preliminary feasibility assessment highlights that although it is legally permissible for DoD and VA to pursue a joint purchased care contract, specific changes to current authorities, regulations, and policies will be required to do so. The specific benefits of an integrated approach to purchasing care with respect to patient experiences (access and quality), as well as the costs to the government, are unclear. Of greatest concern are the significant differences in operational approaches. To achieve desired operational efficiencies from an integrated approach to purchasing care from the private sector, DoD and VA—particularly VA—will need to consider changes to their current operational procedures. Differences in culture, resources, authorities, and budgetary processes will need to be examined closely, and efforts to align them will be necessary. Given the challenges that DoD and VA have previously experienced with increasing resource sharing, we recommend designing and implementing demonstrations or pilots to test the impact of some of these changes before considering more broad-scale changes. As one interviewee commented, "It is not clear that the juice is worth the squeeze." Thus, if DoD and VA leaders remain interested in pursuing an integrated purchased care approach, a pilot program would enable a more careful examination of the impact and potential cost to the government and the U.S. taxpayers before proceeding.

References

Agency for Healthcare Research and Quality, *Evaluating the Impact of Value-Based Purchasing: A Guide for Purchasers*, 2002. As of August 31, 2018:
https://archive.ahrq.gov/professionals/quality-patient-safety/quality-resources/value/valuebased/evalvbp1.html

————, *CAHPS Surveys and Tools to Advance Patient-Centered Care*, 2018. As of August 31, 2018:
https://www.ahrq.gov/cahps/index.html

AHRQ—*See* Agency for Healthcare Research and Quality.

Bagalman, Erin, "The Number of Veterans That Use VA Health Care Services: A Fact Sheet," Washington, D.C.: Congressional Research Service, 2014.

Basu, Sanjay, Jason Andrews, Sandeep Kishore, Rajesh Panjabi, and David Stuckler, "Comparative Performance of Private and Public Healthcare Systems in Low- and Middle-Income Countries: A Systematic Review," *PLOS Medicine*, Vol. 9, No. 6, 2012, e1001244.

Bowen, Deborah J., Matthew Kreuter, Bonnie Spring, Ludmila Cofta-Woerpel, Laura Linnan, Diane Weiner, Suzanne Bakken, Cecilia P. Kaplan, Linda Squiers, Cecilia Fabrizio, and Maria Fernandez, "How We Design Feasibility Studies," *American Journal of Preventive Medicine*, Vol. 36, No. 5, 2009, pp. 452–457.

Burns, Joseph, "HEDIS Is the Hassle That Became a Habit," *Managed Care*, January 14, 2017. As of August 31, 2018:
https://www.managedcaremag.com/archives/2017/1/hedis-hassle-became-habit

CDC—*See* Centers for Disease Control and Prevention.

Centers for Disease Control and Prevention, National Center for Health Statistics, *2013 NCHS Urban–Rural Classification Scheme for Counties*, Vital and Health Statistics, Series 2, Number 166, DHHS Publication No. 2014–1366, 2014. As of August 31, 2018:
https://www.cdc.gov/nchs/data/series/sr_02/sr02_166.pdf

Centers for Medicare and Medicaid Services, "Quality Payment Program," webpage, undated. As of September 24, 2018:
https://qpp.cms.gov/

———, "Original Medicare (Part A and B) Eligibility and Enrollment," webpage, last updated November 3, 2015. As of September 27, 2018:
https://www.cms.gov/Medicare/Eligibility-and-Enrollment/
OrigMedicarePartABEligEnrol/index.html

———, *Medicare Advantage and Section 1876 Cost Plan Network Adequacy Guidance*, February 20, 2018a. As of September 4, 2018:
https://www.cms.gov/Medicare/Medicare-Advantage/MedicareAdvantageApps/
Downloads/2018-Network-Adequacy-Guidance.pdf

———, "Medicare Advantage Applications," webpage, last updated April 2, 2018b. As of September 4, 2018:
https://www.cms.gov/Medicare/Medicare-Advantage/MedicareAdvantageApps/
index.html?redirect=/MedicareAdvantageApps/

———, "The Hospital Value-Based Purchasing (VBP) Program," last updated August 2, 2018c. As of September 24, 2018:
https://www.cms.gov/Medicare/Quality-Initiatives-Patient-Assessment-
Instruments/Value-Based-Programs/HVBP/Hospital-Value-Based-Purchasing.
html

———, "Comprehensive Primary Care Plus," webpage, last updated September 26, 2018d. As of September 27, 2018:
https://innovation.cms.gov/initiatives/Comprehensive-Primary-Care-Plus

Chernew, Michael E., Allison B. Rosen, and A. Mark Fendrick, "Value-Based Insurance Design," *Health Affairs*, Vol. 26, No. 2, March–April 2007, pp. w195–w203.

Chukmaitov, Askar S., David W. Harless, Gloria J. Bazzoli, and Yangyang Deng, "Factors Associated with Hospital Participation in Centers for Medicare and Medicaid Services' Accountable Care Organization Programs," *Health Care Management Review*, September 2017.

CMS—*See* Centers for Medicare and Medicaid Services.

Colla, Carrie H., Valerie A. Lewis, Lee-Sien Kao, A. James O'Malley, Chiang-Hua Chang, and Elliott S. Fisher, "Association Between Medicare Accountable Care Organization Implementation and Spending Among Clinically Vulnerable Beneficiaries," *JAMA Internal Medicine*, Vol. 176, No. 8, 2016, pp. 1167–1175.

Congressional Research Service, *Transfer and Reprogramming of Appropriations: An Overview of Authorities, Limitations, and Procedures*, Washington, D.C., June 6, 2013.

Defense Health Agency, contract with Humana Government Business, No. HT9402-16-C-0001, awarded August 1, 2016.

DHA—*See* Defense Health Agency.

Dworsky, Michael, Carrie M. Farmer, and Mimi Shen, *Veterans' Health Insurance Coverage Under the Affordable Care Act and Implications of Repeal for the Department of Veterans Affairs*, Santa Monica, Calif.: RAND Corporation, RR-1955-NYSHF/RWJ, 2017. As of September 5, 2018:
https://www.rand.org/pubs/research_reports/RR1955.html

Eibner, Christine, Heather Krull, Kristine Brown, Matthew Cefalu, Andrew W. Mulcahy, Michael Pollard, Kanaka Shetty, David M. Adamson, Ernesto F. L. Amaral, Philip Armour, Trinidad Beleche, Olena Bogdan, Jaime L. Hastings, Kandice A. Kapinos, Amii M. Kress, Joshua Mendelsohn, Rachel Ross, Carolyn M. Rutter, Robin M. Weinick, Dulani Woods, Susan D. Hosek, and Carrie M. Farmer, *Current and Projected Characteristics and Unique Health Care Needs of the Patient Population Served by the Department of Veterans Affairs*, Santa Monica, Calif.: RAND Corporation, RR-1165/1-VA, 2015. As of September 5, 2018:
https://www.rand.org/pubs/research_reports/RR1165z1.html

Greenberg, Michael D., Caroline Batka, Christine Buttorff, Molly Dunigan, Susan L. Lovejoy, Geoffrey McGovern, Nicholas M. Pace, Francesca Pillemer, Kayla M. Williams, Eric Apaydin, Clara Aranibar, Maya Buenaventura, Phillip Carter, Samantha Cherney, Lynn E. Davis, Amy Grace Donohue, Lily Geyer, Joslyn Fleming, Parisa Roshan, Lauren Skrabala, Stephen Simmons, Joseph Thompson, Jonathan Welch, Susan D. Hosek, and Carrie M. Farmer, *Authorities and Mechanisms for Purchased Care at the Department of Veterans Affairs*, Santa Monica, Calif.: RAND Corporation, RR-1165/3-VA, 2015. As of August 31, 2018:
https://www.rand.org/pubs/research_reports/RR1165z3.html

Gruber, Jonathan, and Robin McKnight, "Controlling Health Care Costs Through Limited Network Insurance Plans: Evidence from Massachusetts State Employees," *American Economic Journal: Economic Policy*, Vol. 8, No. 2, 2016, pp. 219–250.

Henry J. Kaiser Family Foundation, *Health Costs: 2017 Employer Health Benefits Survey*, September 19, 2017. As of September 4, 2018:
https://www.kff.org/health-costs/report/2017-employer-health-benefits-survey

Hepner, Kimberly A., Carol P. Roth, Elizabeth M. Sloss, Susan M. Paddock, Praise O. Iyiewuare, Martha J. Timmer, and Harold Alan Pincus, *Quality of Care for PTSD and Depression in the Military Health System: Final Report*, Santa Monica, Calif.: RAND Corporation, RR-1542-OSD, 2017. As of September 5, 2018:
https://www.rand.org/pubs/research_reports/RR1542.html

Hebert, Paul L., Adam S. Batten, Eric Gunnink, Ashok Reddy, Edwin S. Wong, Stephan D. Fihn, and Chuan-Fen Liu, "Reliance on Medicare Providers by Veterans After Becoming Age-Eligible for Medicare Is Associated with the Use of More Outpatient Services," *Health Services Research*, special issue, September 2018.

Hsu, John, Mary Price, Jenna Spirt, Christine Vogeli, Richard Brand, Michael E. Chernew, Sreekanth K. Chaguturu, Namita Mohta, Eric Weil, and Timothy Ferris, "Patient Population Loss at a Large Pioneer Accountable Care Organization and Implications for Refining the Program," *Health Affairs*, Vol. 35, No. 3, March 2016, pp. 422–430.

Huang, Grace, Benjamin Muz, Sharon Kim, and Joseph Gasper, *2017 Survey of Veteran Enrollees' Health and Use of Health Care: Data Findings Report*, Rockville, Md.: Westat, April 2018. As of September 5, 2018:
https://www.va.gov/HEALTHPOLICYPLANNING/SoE2017/VA_Enrollees_Report_Data_Findings_Report2.pdf

KFF—*See* Henry J. Kaiser Family Foundation.

Kizer, Kenneth, John G. Demakis, and John R. Feussner, "Reinventing VA Health Care: Systematizing Quality Improvement and Quality Innovation," *Medical Care*, Vol. 38, No. 6, June 2000, pp. I-7–I-16.

Kizer, Kenneth, and R. Adams Dudley, "Extreme Makeover: Transformation of the Veterans Health Care System," *Annual Review of Public Health*, Vol. 30, 2009, pp. 313–339.

Miles, Donna, "TRICARE to Extend Dependent Coverage to Age 26," American Forces Press Service, January 14, 2011. As of September 27, 2018:
http://www.navy.mil/submit/display.asp?story_id=58052

Military Health System, "About the Military Health System," webpage, undated(a). As of August 31, 2018:
http://www.health.mil/About-MHS

———, "Annual Evaluation of the TRICARE Program," webpage, undated(b). As of September 4, 2018:
https://www.health.mil/Military-Health-Topics/Access-Cost-Quality-and-Safety/Health-Care-Program-Evaluation/Annual-Evaluation-of-the-TRICARE-Program

———, "CMAC Rates," webpage, undated(c). As of September 4, 2018:
https://health.mil/Military-Health-Topics/Business-Support/Rates-and-Reimbursement/CMAC-Rates

———, homepage, undated(d). As of August 31, 2018:
https://health.mil

———, "Joint Incentive Fund," webpage, undated(e). As of October 17, 2018:
https://www.health.mil/Military-Health-Topics/Access-Cost-Quality-and-Safety/Access-to-Healthcare/DoD-VA-Sharing-Initiatives/Joint-Resource-Sharing/JIF

———, "MHS GENESIS," webpage, undated(f). As of September 4, 2018:
https://health.mil/mhsgenesis

Mulcahy, Andrew W., Italo A. Gutierrez, Tadeja Gracner, Teague Ruder, George E. Hart, and Melony E. Sorbero, *The Impact of Health Reform on Purchased Care Access: National Health Reform and Modernization of the Military Health System Study*, Santa Monica, Calif.: RAND Corporation, RR-1627-OSD, 2017. As of September 19, 2018:
https://www.rand.org/pubs/research_reports/RR1627.html

NCQA—*See* National Committee for Quality Assurance.

National Committee for Quality Assurance, "HEDIS and Performance Measurement," webpage, undated. As of September 27, 2018:
https://www.ncqa.org/hedis

———, *NCQA Health Insurance Plan Ratings*, 2017. As of August 31, 2018:
http://www.ncqa.org/report-cards/health-plans/health-insurance-plan-ratings/ncqa-health-insurance-plan-ratings-2017

Nyweide, David J., Woolton Lee, Timothy T. Cuerdon, Hoangmai H. Pham, Megan Cox, Rahul Rajkumar, and Patrick H. Conway, "Association of Pioneer Accountable Care Organizations vs Traditional Medicare Fee for Service with Spending, Utilization, and Patient Experience," *Journal of the American Medical Association*, Vol. 313, No. 21, June 2, 2015, pp. 2152–2161.

Panangala, Sidath Viranga, *Health Care for Veterans: Answers to Frequently Asked Questions*, Washington, D.C.: Congressional Research Service, April 21, 2016.

Philpott, Tom, "New TRICARE Contracts Shake Up Fees for Some Startled Doctors," *Daily Press*, May 7, 2017. As of September 5, 2018:
http://www.dailypress.com/news/military/dp-nws-military-update-0508-20170507-story.html

Public Law 104-262, Veterans' Health Care Eligibility Reform Act of 1996, October 9, 1996.

Public Law 107-314, Bob Stump National Defense Authorization Act for Fiscal Year 2003, December 2, 2002.

Public Law 113-146, Veterans Access, Choice and Accountability Act of 2014, August 7, 2014.

Public Law 114-328, National Defense Authorization Act for Fiscal Year 2017, December 23, 2016.

Public Law 115-97, Tax Cuts and Jobs Act, December 22, 2017.

Public Law 115-141, Consolidated Appropriations Act, 2018, March 23, 2018.

Public Law 115-182, VA Maintaining Systems and Strengthening Integrated Outside Networks (MISSION) Act of 2018, June 6, 2018.

Public Law 115-232, John S. McCain National Defense Authorization Act for Fiscal Year 2019, August 13, 2018.

Public Law 115-244, Energy and Water, Legislative Branch, and Military Construction and Veterans Affairs Appropriations Act, 2019, September 21, 2018.

Robinson, James C., Christopher M. Whaley, and Timothy T. Brown. "Association of Reference Pricing with Drug Selection and Spending," *New England Journal of Medicine*, Vol. 377, No. 7, 2017, pp. 658–665.

Robinson, James C., Timothy T. Brown, and Christopher Whaley, "Reference Pricing Changes The 'Choice Architecture' Of Health Care for Consumers." *Health Affairs*, Vol. 36, No. 3, 2017, pp. 524–530.

Rostker, Bernard, *Providing for the Casualties of War: The American Experience Through World War II*, Santa Monica, Calif.: RAND Corporation, MG-1164-OSD, 2013. As of August 14, 2018: https://www.rand.org/pubs/monographs/MG1164.html

Severo, Richard, and Lewis Milford, *The Wages of War: When America's Soldiers Came Home—From Valley Forge to Vietnam*, New York: Simon and Schuster, 1989.

Tanielian, Terri, Carrie M. Farmer, Rachel M. Burns, Erin L. Duffy, and Claude Messan Setodji, *Ready or Not? Assessing the Capacity of New York State Health Care Providers to Meet the Needs of Veterans*, Santa Monica, Calif.: RAND Corporation, RR-2298-NYSHF, 2018. As of September 5, 2018: https://www.rand.org/pubs/research_reports/RR2298.html

Tollestrup, Jessica, *Advance Appropriations, Forward Funding, and Advance Funding: Concepts, Practice, and Budget Process Considerations*, Washington, D.C.: Congressional Research Service, October 8, 2015.

TRICARE, "Continued Health Care Benefit Program," webpage, undated(a). As of September 27, 2018: https://www.tricare.mil/Plans/SpecialPrograms/CHCBP

———, "Transitional Assistance Management Program," webpage, undated(b). As of September 5, 2018: https://tricare.mil/Plans/SpecialPrograms/TAMP

———, "TRICARE Mental Health Care Services Fact Sheet," 2016. As of August 31, 2018: http://www.tricare.mil/~/media/Files/TRICARE/Publications/FactSheets/Mental_Health_FS.pdf

———, *TRICARE for Life Handbook*, March 2018a. As of August 31, 2018: https://www.tricare.mil/~/media/Files/TRICARE/Publications/Handbooks/TFL_HBK.pdf

———, *January 2018 Health Care Survey of DoD Beneficiaries*, 2018b. As of September 6, 2018: https://tricare.mil/survey/hcsdbsurvey/home/z_abr_form.cfm

U.S. Department of Defense, *TRICARE Management Activity Report to Congress on TRICARE's Physician Reimbursement Rates and Their Adequacy*, Washington, D.C., February 2007. As of September 5, 2018:
https://health.mil/Reference-Center/Reports/2007/02/05/Physician-Reimbursement-Rates-and-Their-Adequacy

———, *Military Health System Review: Final Report to the Secretary of Defense*, Washington, D.C., August 2014. As of September 5, 2018:
https://archive.defense.gov/pubs/140930_MHS_Review_Final_Report_Main_Body.pdf

———, *Evaluation of the TRICARE Program: Access, Cost, and Quality—Fiscal Year 2015 Report to Congress*, Washington, D.C., 2015. As of August 31, 2018:
https://www.health.mil/Reference-Center/Reports/2015/02/28/Evaluation-of-the-TRICARE-Program-Fiscal-Year-2015-Report-to-Congress

———, *Report to the Armed Services Committees on Pilot Program on Incorporation of Value-Based Health Care in Purchased Care Component of TRICARE Program and Report on Implementation Plan—Value-Based Incentives/Managed Care Support Contract Strategy for TRICARE*, Washington, D.C., 2017.

———, *Evaluation of the TRICARE Program: Fiscal Year 2018 Report to Congress*, Washington, D.C., February 28, 2018. As of October 17, 2018:
https://www.health.mil/Military-Health-Topics/Access-Cost-Quality-and-Safety/Health-Care-Program-Evaluation/Annual-Evaluation-of-the-TRICARE-Program

U.S. Department of Defense, Office of the Actuary, *Valuation of the Military Retirement System*, September 2016. As of September 5, 2018:
https://media.defense.gov/2018/Jun/08/2001928794/-1/-1/0/MRF%20VALRPT%202016%20[JUNE%202018].PDF

U.S. Department of Defense Financial Management Regulation, Vol. 11A, Reimbursable Operations Policy, Ch. 3, Economy Act Order, current as of March 2012. As of October 17, 2018:
https://comptroller.defense.gov/Portals/45/documents/fmr/Volume_11a.pdf

U.S. Department of Defense Instruction 6010.23, *DoD and Department of Veterans Affairs (VA) Health Care Resource Sharing Program*, October 3, 2013.

U.S. Department of Veterans Affairs, *Community Care Network (CCN), RFP for Services*, Solicitation Number VA79116R0086, December 2016a.

———, *Eligibility for and Enrollment in VA Healthcare*, 2016b. As of August 31, 2018:
http://www.mentalhealth.va.gov/communityproviders/docs/Eligibility_Criteria.pdf

———, "Enrollment Priority Groups," fact sheet, December 2016c. As of September 27, 2018:
https://www.va.gov/healthbenefits/resources/publications/IB10-441_enrollment_priority_groups.pdf

————, "About VHA," webpage 2017a. As of August 31, 2018:
https://www.va.gov/health/aboutVHA.asp

————, *Department of Veterans Affairs: Budget in Brief 2017*, 2017b.

————, *Veterans Health Administration, VA Monograph, Office of Information and Technology, Enterprise Program Management Office, and Office of Information and Analytics*, 2017c. As of September 4, 2018:
https://www.va.gov/VISTA_MONOGRAPH/VA_Monograph.pdf

————, *Veterans Choice Program (VCP) Provider Satisfaction Survey*, 2017d.

————, "Organizational Chart and Full-Time Employment Numbers (FTE)," 2018a.

————, Volume II, *Medical Programs and Information Technology Programs, Congressional Submission, FY 2019 Funding and FY 2020 Advance Appropriations*, 2018b. As of August 31, 2018:
https://www.va.gov/budget/docs/summary/
fy2019VAbudgetVolumeIImedicalProgramsAndInformationTechnology.pdf

Veterans of Foreign Wars, *Our Care 2017: A Report Evaluating Veterans Health Care*, 2017. As of September 4, 2018:
https://www.vfw.org/vawatch

VFW—*See* Veterans of Foreign Wars.

Wehrwein, Peter, "Pioneer ACOS: And Then There Were 23," *Managed Care*, September 28, 2013. As of August 31, 2018:
https://www.managedcaremag.com/archives/2013/9/
pioneer-acos-and-then-there-were-23